Kate Cook's
Wellness
Guide

Inspiring health choices
for your well-being
transformation

infiniteideas

Copyright © Infinite Ideas 2013, 2017

The right of Kate Cook to be identified as the author of this book has been asserted in accordance with the Copyright, Designs and Patents Act 1988.

First published in 2013 as *The corporate wellness bible* by
Infinite Ideas Limited
36 St Giles
Oxford
OX1 3LD
United Kingdom
www.infideas.com

This edition published 2017

A CIP catalogue record for this book is available from the British Library

ISBN 978–1–908984–91–3

Contents

**Part 3: Exercise your way to Wellness
(even if you think you don't have the time)**

Part 4: Wellness – it's all in the mind

Foreword

As our lives move ever faster, it can sometimes feel that from the start to the end of the day is all a bit of a blur. Every day we're a little bit more stressed, having to work that little bit longer, and we're starting to lose our cool just that little bit more frequently.

Many of us find it difficult to eat healthily these days and the main reason is time – we're always in a hurry. We're not making time for breakfast, even lunch becomes a bit of a luxury, and we find ourselves trying to make up for it with an overly large dinner, far too late in the evening.

We also experience sleep problems. It's difficult to take time to relax when you're rushing between work, the kids' after school clubs and the supermarket and still trying to have a social life. Many of us even feel guilty about relaxing. Whatever the cause, sleep problems are on the rise, and many of us find that when we get to bed we're not yet ready to sleep, as our minds are still fully focused on the unfinished business of today and the tough challenges we need to prepare for tomorrow.

We're constantly told that we should exercise more if we want to avoid common health problems so we dutifully sign up for the gym, full of good intentions. But a few months into the year the gym membership card is gathering dust and our determined New Year resolutions have gone by the by – we are just too frenetically busy.

Recognising that cutting out the commute may be the way to salvage a few hours, some of us have tried working from home. This tactic initially appears to pay off but many of us have discovered that the extra commuting hour gets lost as we just work even longer hours. Worse still work's always there in the background, nagging at us. To top it all we still can't make time for lunch.

Now, we all realise that holidays are important and a great way to unwind (though the credit crunch dealt a savage blow to them). Unfortunately we're often too busy to think about organising them and even when we have booked them way in advance we're often still rushing around at the last minute trying to finish all our work before we jet off. We might well end up booking and leaving in a bit of a mad rush because we didn't make the time to organise everything and pack properly. By the time we reach our destination we're absolutely frazzled and it takes us the best part of a week to relax enough to enjoy ourselves. Before we know it we're back home and back on the treadmill again.

If we don't take the time to address the situation all this busyness and stress just accumulates, taking its inevitable toll on our health, relationships and appearance. It's easy to carry on this way just thinking that's how your life's going to be. If we're 'lucky' something will shock us out of our routine; perhaps a friend our age has a stroke or finds their marriage has collapsed around their ears. We look at the friend's lifestyle and realise we're not that different; we see where our crazy, rushed, disorganised life is leading.

So it's time to take a little time out for ourselves on a regular basis. Well-being and Wellness are not fads, they're essential to a better way of life.

Since meeting Kate Cook, she has transformed how I think and feel about my health; and I'm not the only one she's helped. In this book, Kate leads us through a fun and easy guide for better and healthier living. Kate never lectures, and she never tells you off; what she does do is encourage you to take things into your own hands. Her easy-to-read and simple-to-follow guidelines really do make you want to help yourself and believe you can do it. Kate is fun, witty and always instructive. Start the first day to a better life here and encourage your friends and family to join in too – this is not a book for keeping to yourself but for sharing with those you care about.

Kate has made a tangible difference to many individuals, to many teams and many organisations; it's time for her to help you to help yourself as well.

Rene Carayol

Introduction

You are holding a precious gift in your hands – the key to Wellness. As they say, 'health is wealth'! Without health all our hard work, freedoms, relationships and money can't be enjoyed: it's all worthless.

This book is designed for those of us who work and sometimes compromise health for long hours and bad habits. Work is where we spend a *lot* of our time – so we need to practise Wellness at work on a regular basis or there just won't be enough time once you get home. Slow and steady change is what we are after. Of course everyone has days where good intentions fly out of the window – that's just human. So no 'waggy-finger' telling you off here but a book stuffed full of easy-to-digest suggestions (sorry – no pun intended).

I've divided the book into four sections. In the first you can identify your particular health concerns and find some pointers towards chapters that might help you. The other three sections are crammed with ideas on diet, exercise and the psychology of Wellness. The idea is that you can just dip into the book, reading the chapter most helpful to you at the time, though by all means if you want to read it from cover to cover, be my guest. The book is accessible and easy to read and will provide you with some effective yet simple (and often small) actions you can take when starting on your health and Wellness journey. Some stuff you will ignore and some stuff you will think is a good idea and it will spark something off inside you and gradually, almost without you noticing, you will start to change.

As a nutritionist I would suggest that you start with diet as a foundation, but really wherever you feel most comfortable beginning your voyage will be the right place for you. Change is rarely revolutionary – most change is an organic process over a period of time. So give yourself a pat on the back for being on the road and see where it takes you.

If you want vibrant energy this book is a great place to start … so get stuck in!

Please do keep in touch! I would love to hear your stories.

Go well and good health

Kate

kate@katecook.biz

Acknowledgement

I'd like to thank Kevin Nind (MSc) for his contributions to chapters 5, 8, 11, 45, 73, 79 and for the boxes on pages 92, 267, 275, 276, 328 and 332. Kevin is an occupational psychologist and associate fellow with the British Psychological Society as well as a registered psychologist with the Health and Care Professions Council. He has a long-standing interest in promoting a healthy approach to work, by helping organisations become better places to work and enabling individuals to thrive even in pressured environments. Through his extensive knowledge of psychological research, tools, techniques and practical exercises, Kevin has developed workshops, events and courses on stress management, and resilience for numerous organisations.

Part 1

Is your Wellness under threat?

We all have obstacles that stop us living our lives to their fullest. Whether your issues are health related, to do with your finances or just about making more time, read on to find out why it's important to address them. Whether you spring out of bed with a smile on your face at 6 o'clock every morning or find the daily routine a bit more of a struggle, start by taking our helpful quiz to discover what changes you might need to make.

Work out your Wellness score

Do you have good lifestyle, exercise and eating habits? Be honest now. We understand that it's difficult to be good all the time and can seem quite dull. Rules about fruit and veg portions and BMI guidelines may not be sexy, but put all those 'dull' recommendations together and you have the holy grail of Wellness, a recipe for energy and *joie de vivre*.

The truth is, it's never to early to start listening to your body, and doing right by it. The aim of the following questionnaire is to encourage you to do some proper soul-searching about how much respect you have for that body of yours, and start thinking about what you can do today to boost your Wellness tomorrow and beyond.

Decide whether each of the statements below is largely true or false for you.

1. I get at least seven hours sleep a night at least five days a week.

2. When it comes to snacking, the fruit bowl holds more appeal for me than the cake tin – I can't get enough of those antioxidants.

3. I exercise for at least half an hour three days a week.

4. I take a multivitamin/supplement every day.

5. I get lots of relaxation every day – meditation, yoga, taking time out is really good for my stress levels.

6. My parents are still fighting fit, or lived to a ripe old age.

7. (Women) I'm up to date with all my smear tests.

8. (Men) I'm not too embarrassed to check my testicles regularly.

9. I get at least nine portions of fruit and veg a day.

10. I regularly give my liver a rest – alcohol-free days are a must.

11. My body fat percentage is within healthy limits.

12. I try not to eat meat more than a couple of times a week and stick to fish or poultry.

13. I don't say no to the odd indulgence, but fortunately I'm the kind of person who knows how to stop.

14. I always have my regular dentist check-up.

15. If I need to shift pounds, I tend to do it slowly and steadily – I'm not a binge eater and would never starve myself.

16. I drink 6 to 8 glasses of water a day – more when I'm exercising or drinking alcohol.

17. I get plenty of omega 3 oils, such as those from oily fish, in my diet.

18. I get my blood pressure checked regularly – and it's within healthy limits.

19. I do everything I can to stay as healthy as possible.

Award yourself one point for each time you answer 'true' to a question.

Score

16–19 points

Top marks. Sounds like you're as au fait with good health and nutrition as a person can be. You're probably vegan, teetotal and never binge on anything more decadent than alfafa sprouts. Don't forget that moderation is also a pretty good path to follow – when it comes to health, those who border on the fanatical don't win many friends. But then again, you may live longer, so I suppose you get the last laugh ...

10–16 points

Mr or Ms Average – chances are your intentions are good – you're eating well, exercising regularly-ish, and it appears you do strive to stay on the right side of healthy. As long as your good, healthy habits outweigh the bad, you'll be winning. But remember, the key is to find a balance between saintly and sinful behaviour.

Under 10

Oh dear, oh dear, oh dear – got a deathwish or something? All that partying and indulgence may seem good for your well-being right now, but remember, it's easy to believe you're immortal when you're a youngster. The truth is sooner or later you've got to wise up to the benefits of drinking plenty of water, getting those health checks done, waking up to the power of exercise, and welcoming into your lifestyle all those elements which will help keep you in rude health well into your twilight years. Read on ... concentrate ... and prepare to turn over a new leaf.

Most of us know the basics of what we should do to be well. Few of us do it. That's just a fact. Unfortunately there are no short cuts if you're not addressing the basics. These include:

- eating enough good-quality food to provide your cells with energy and keep energy production strong and constant;

- drinking enough fluids to remain hydrated;

- sleeping enough to restore your body;

- learning how to relax;

- maintaining a sensible work–life balance;

- exercising enough to keep your lungs and heart functioning healthily and pumping blood to your cells, where it supplies the nutrients you need; and

- stopping the really bad habits such as smoking, binge drinking and drug taking.

Perhaps you used to have all this under control. Perhaps you're a mother who just hasn't time to eat properly or exercise, and are undergoing sleep disruption; perhaps work has got frantic over the last six months and you're so stressed you can't be bothered to look after yourself; perhaps your job demands a lot of travel – if you travel a lot, it's well-nigh impossible to take care of the basics unless you put some good systems in place and stick to them until they're habits. The good news is that there are lots of short cuts that will help you and easy ways to get your basics in place. First of all though let's take a look at the most common problems that can affect your health and well-being.

1

A weighty issue
(or, a weighty question)

Judging by the newspaper headlines screaming about some new statistic or research about obesity, you'd think there was a moral obligation to be thin.

Often the subtext is that fat people get sick and are a burden on our medical resources. And then there are the images of super-slim models and celebrities that confront us in magazines and on our TV and movie screens. The underlying message here is that this is the way you're supposed to look, especially if you want to be happy and successful, not to mention being sexually attractive. There are more overweight than starving people on the planet and unfortunately that's not because we've solved the world's hunger problems. It's enough to make you choke on your chocolate bar, isn't it?

Obesity is undeniably a growing problem in the Western world, due mainly to the over-consumption of the wrong kinds of foods and decreased activity levels. Experts warn of the host of health dangers to which carrying too much weight exposes you, including heart disease, diabetes, high blood pressure and, for women in particular (though not exclusively), fertility problems. It's not guaranteed that you'll develop these kinds of health problems – obesity just heightens your risk, which is of course why most of us just carry on regardless – until something goes wrong. The chances are that if you're already suffering any of the conditions mentioned, your doctor has grilled you on your diet and suggested losing weight.

For the majority of us, slimming down is more of a preventative health measure or something we want to do for cosmetic reasons: i.e. we just don't like the way we look. This is fine, as long as it isn't interfering with daily life and manifesting itself as disordered eating (anorexia, bulimia, faddy eating and so on). If that is the case for you, please seek help through a doctor or therapist. Life is too short and too precious not to enjoy it to the full.

Working out if you're really overweight is easily done using the Body Mass Index calculation. The BMI is far from perfect, so it is not without its critics (partly because if you're quite well-muscled, you'll be heavy, not fat, because muscle weighs more than fat) but you have to start somewhere! All you have to do is weigh yourself and record the result in kilograms. Then measure your height in metres. Then do the following sum[*]:

weight in kilograms divided by (height in metres × height in metres) = BMI

Example:

> You weigh 70 kg and you are 1.6 metres tall
>
> $70 \div (1.6 \times 1.6) =$
>
> $70 \div 2.56 = 27.34$
>
> BMI = 27.34

Check your own result against the ranges below

BMI for men	BMI for women	
Under 20	under 19	underweight
20–24.9	19–24.9	normal
25–29.9	25–29.9	overweight
30 plus	30 plus	obese

Many experts are now saying that abdominal fat is the killer, with apple-shaped people who have relatively slim hips and a larger waist being more at risk from developing heart disease than the pear-shaped – those who carry their fat on their hips and thighs. The ideal waist measurement for men is less than 95 cm (37 inches) and less than 80 cm (32 inches) for women. Over 100 cm (40 inches) for a man and over 90 cm (35 inches) for a woman indicates the greatest risk to health.

We can blame our parents for lots of things, including a tendency to gain weight. However, much of 'hereditary' weight gain can also be explained by learned behaviour. For instance, if you come from a family that loves food, overeating may be part of your lifestyle, but habits can be unlearned.

Your RMR, or resting metabolic rate, is the number of calories your body needs to maintain its vital functions. This is partly to do with genetic inheritance. A friend who is a similar height and weight to you may well be able to eat more than you and not gain weight. This is very annoying, but you're probably better at other things than he or she is. Human beings are not boilers so we all process our food resources differently, depending on a range of factors. Pure calorie calculations only provide a basic guide. There are two other things to remember. First, if you have less body fat and more muscle, your metabolism will be higher, as muscle burns up more calories than fat. That's why including exercise in your weight loss plan really works. Second, don't try to cut calories drastically, as your metabolic rate will slow to adjust – and you'll just feel hungry all the time. Eating less but eating well is the key to long-term weight loss.

Does being overweight really matter?

Suppose that you realise that you are overweight. Perhaps you have not got back into shape after having children or maybe you have always been a little plumper than you would like. Is it really a problem?

A few curves and a couple of extra kilos can be flattering and sensual – and that goes for men as well as women. So when does a little plumpness become unacceptable? It depends on your viewpoint. If carrying a few extra kilos doesn't bother you, then it is not a health issue. If it annoys you because you want to be in better shape, or it diminishes your confidence or stops you wearing the clothes you want to wear, then maybe you should do something about it. If you have more than a few extra kilos, it does start to matter and when you're properly overweight it starts to matter very much indeed.

In 2014, just over a quarter of adults (25.6 per cent of people aged 16 or over) in England were classified as obese. Alarmingly children are getting larger too – for the same period, around three in ten boys and girls (aged 2 to 15) were classed as either overweight or obese.

Obesity makes everyday life uncomfortable is so many ways, such as being unable to run for a bus, a lack of choice in clothes, rude stares and comments from other, thinner, people, and sleep and fertility problems. It is also the commonest cause of ill health and potentially fatal diseases. Obesity contributes to heart disease, diabetes, gallstones and some cancers. Just being overweight – and that's more than say a kilo or so – can raise your blood pressure and give you health problems. Even dental decay is more common in overweight people.

In case you're in any doubt as to why being overweight does matter, here are some fat facts to consider:

According to the British Heart Foundation, heart and circulatory disease is the UK's biggest killer. Although the numbers are in fact slightly lower than twenty years ago, this is because of medical advances, not because we are getting healthier! There are other risk factors too, such as smoking, poor psychological health and inherited infirmities, but the truth is that 30 per cent of deaths from coronary heart disease are directly linked to an unhealthy diet.

What about fasting?

One diet that has been gaining a lot of good publicity recently is the Fast (or 5:2) Diet. It may sound like a fad but research is lending weight to the theory that eating a reduced diet two days per week and eating normally the rest of the time can improve both your health and your waistline and even increase your lifespan. In *The Fast Diet: The Secret of Intermittent Fasting – Lose Weight, Stay Healthy, Live Longer*, Mimi Spencer and Dr Michael Mosley claim that the fasting works by preventing your body from going into fat-storage mode. In prehistoric times when food couldn't be stored we weren't always able to eat every day and so the body is used to intermittent fasting. And by giving your body time to recover from processing food on the 'fast days' you enable it to repair itself.

The World Health Organization estimates that somewhere between 1 and 24 per cent of coronary heart disease is due to doing less than two and a half hours of moderate activity a week.

The fatter you are, the greater your risk. A weight gain of just 10 kg doubles your risk of heart disease. If you are apple-shaped, with more fat around your middle, your risk of heart disease is greater than if you're pear-shaped, with more fat on your bottom. Divide your waist measurement by your hip measurement (in centimetres). If the result is more than 0.95 for a man or 0.87 for a woman, you are apple-shaped.

Excess weight plays a part in high blood pressure, which can lead to blood clots, stroke and heart attacks. You can reduce these risks through diet: less processed food, which tends to be higher in salt, a huge increase in fruit and vegetable consumption and eating healthy fat, such as the omega-3s found principally in fish.

Although the exact relationships are not fully understood, diet and cancer have an association too. A recent report suggested that as many as 40 per cent of cancers have a dietary link. Breast cancer risk rises with a high fat diet or being overweight.

Clearly there's still a lot of research to be done, but it is certain that being overweight isn't fun and it isn't clever – and it can be about a lot more than the way you look.

You might find chapters 25, 26, 28, 30 and 45 especially helpful.

2
Could you have diabetes?

Diabetes is increasing on a global scale. Even more concerning is the fact that you could be a sufferer without knowing it. Currently (November 2016) almost 3.6 million people in the UK have been diagnosed with diabetes, with an estimated further million undiagnosed. By 2025 it is estimated that over 4 million people in the UK will be diagnosed diabetic. The majority of these cases (roughly 90 per cent) are Type 2 diabetes.

Diabetes is not new – in the seventeenth century it was called the 'pissing evil' – but it is on the increase. There are two types of diabetes. Type 1 is more commonly found in children and young adults and is treated with a strict diet and insulin injections. It's Type 2 that is on the increase and is strongly linked to obesity and a lack of activity. There are other risk factors over which we have no control, such as genetic inheritance, simply getting older and your ethnic origin – people from Asian and Afro-Caribbean backgrounds do seem to be at a higher risk. Eating lots of sweet things, contrary to popular belief, doesn't directly cause diabetes, but it leads to weight gain, which does increase your risk. It's a fact that 80 per cent of people with Type 2 diabetes are overweight. The fatter and less fit you are, the greater your risk.

Type 2 diabetes used to be more common in middle age, but increasingly it's affecting younger people too. Those with the condition either don't produce enough insulin or what is produced doesn't work effectively, which means that the body can't use glucose properly and levels remain high in the blood. Some of the symptoms of undiagnosed diabetes include increased thirst, a need to go to the toilet often, especially at night, lethargy and tiredness, blurred vision, regular thrush and genital itching, plus weight loss when nothing else has changed regarding your lifestyle. Doctors say many people have these symptoms on and off for years before eventually being diagnosed as diabetic, which is easily done with a simple blood test.

The World Health Organization thinks Type 2 diabetes is a big issue. It is predicting a global epidemic of diabetes, which means that it already is an issue for you and it will definitely be an issue for your children. In many developing countries, people are getting diabetes at a staggering rate because they eat all the newly available refined foods. How many people do you know who have diabetes? Why don't you ask them what they think about this? You might be very surprised at their response.

In the past, if you were diagnosed as having diabetes, physical activity was discouraged and a high fat/low carbohydrate diet prescribed. Now exercise is encouraged, just as it is for everyone to improve their health and control their weight. As a role model, look to Sir Steve Redgrave, five times Olympic Gold medal winner and a diabetes sufferer! Diet-wise, the reason a high fat diet was recommended was to make up for the lack of calories that resulted from following a low carbohydrate diet to keep sugar levels stable (fat doesn't boost sugar levels in itself). In recent years this approach has made a redurgence. Obviously, keeping refined carbohydrate intake to a minimum is vital and most diabetics can control their condition and also lose weight by eating in the most healthful way. Diabetics also need to ensure that any medicine they are taking is monitored by their doctor.

Four out of five people with the condition die prematurely from heart disease. Action is essential, both if you've already been diagnosed and also as a preventative measure. Do ask your doctor for a test if any of the risk factors apply to you and also if you have any of the symptoms described above. This is definitely not a disease you want to get, and so many of us can fend it off by keeping our bodies healthy.

You might find chapters 15 and 16 and the box on page 73 especially helpful.

3

Control your blood pressure

So you're 120 over 80. Or maybe you're 140 over 90. Be honest, do you really know what that means?

You've had your blood pressure checked. The doctor 'hmm's and says, 'That's fine.' You take a deep breath and ask, 'What is it?' Slowly your doctor raises her head and looks you straight in the eye.

Smiling nervously, you're just about to tell her that it really doesn't matter, feeling you've crossed the line, when she smiles and says, 120 over 80. Sighing you say great, OK, thank you, and leave as quickly as possible.

Two minutes later as you're enjoying the moment the anti-climax hits you head-on. 120 over 80. My blood pressure is 120 over 80. So what? You've little idea what this means. It's another number to add to the list. Twenty-twenty vision, body mass index of 24, a perfect ten, and now 120 over 80.

The heart is basically a muscle whose job is to pump blood around the body. Blood is pumped from the heart, it travels around the body delivering oxygen and nutrients to the organs of the body, and returns to the heart ready to be pumped back out again. It's like a water pump in a garden water feature. To work the heart needs a power supply, and this is electrical. So the heart is an electrical, muscular pump.

An adult has around five litres of blood that circulates around the body approximately once every minute. As the blood passes through your arteries, the force it exerts on the artery walls is your blood pressure.

The top figure, called the systolic blood pressure, is the pressure in blood vessels when the heart is pumping blood out. The lower figure, called the diastolic pressure, is the pressure in blood vessels when the heart is filling with blood again. The heart contracts, or squeezes, so blood is pushed out into the circulation, then it relaxes. So squeeze and relax, squeeze and relax.

OK, so you now know what the two blood pressure figures represent. But what you really want to know is what is normal. It's often said that 120 over 80 is the 'normal' blood pressure. The reality is that there's a range of readings that will be considered 'normal', or better still, safe, which is why doctors go on and on about blood pressure. If your blood pressure becomes too high a whole range of nasties like heart attacks and strokes can shorten your life. High blood pressure will cost you financially too: insurance premiums, for example, are likely to be higher. Moreover, high blood pressure invariably doesn't cause any symptoms, so the first time people learn they have hypertension (the medical term for high blood pressure) is when something does blow, often with tragic consequences. And that's why having it checked is important.

Both the upper and lower figures are important. In the past it was the lower figure that was believed to be most important. Now it's agreed that whether the top figure, or lower figure, or both figures are high, treatment to bring these raised readings down to a safe level is a very good idea since doing this will reduce the risk of future health problems such as heart failure, heart attacks and stroke.

In years gone by when less was known and understood about blood pressure 100 plus your age was accepted as a safe upper limit for systolic pressure. But now we know better (until the science changes again). The accumulated wisdom of scientific research has concluded that having a blood pressure reading that is less than 140/90 is desirable. If you have high blood pressure or other medical conditions your doctor will probably have told you that it is desirable for your blood pressure to be even less than this.

Like the value of investments blood pressure can go up as well as down – so what causes those changes? Which ones should have you worried?

With blood pressure, happiness is a blood pressure that may go up temporarily but spends most of its time out of the danger zone.

Of course blood pressure that is too low isn't desirable either. You've watched the medical dramas on TV and heard a tense nurse exclaim, 'Pressure's dropping, 80 over 40.' The look on her face and on the faces around her tell you this is not good. In fact you don't need to be told, because one look at the guy on the table says, this really isn't good. But it's high blood pressure that is generally considered to be an everyday problem.

Blood pressure goes up and down throughout the day. If you run up the stairs or run for the bus, your blood pressure goes up. Overnight while you're asleep, it goes down. This is normal. So relax. These fluctuations are temporary, which makes them fine. The meeting with the boss, presentations in public, having the in-laws to stay, all can cause your blood pressure to rise. As James Bond lay on the table and Goldfinger's laser crept slowly towards his vital parts, you can bet your bottom dollar his blood pressure was rising.

These increases in blood pressure are good. They are a normal response of the body. They are also temporary, which is important. It's when blood pressure is consistently high that things get a little twitchy. High blood pressure generally doesn't cause symptoms, so you wouldn't know your blood pressure was high. Not until it was measured, or disaster struck.

For around nine out of ten people with high blood pressure there is no underlying cause. Years of good, but less than healthy living, would have contributed to the level rising above the 140/90 ceiling. The bottom line: pressure that is consistently above this level is bad news. Without appropriate intervention there's a risk you are going to crash. If your blood pressure is looking inflated, you have to adjust your risk factors. This means less salt (especially abundant in processed food), alcohol and weight, and more activity, fruit and vegetables. You can't change who you are, but you can change what you are.

You might find chapters 49, 50 and 56 especially helpful.

4

Daily habits – smoking and drinking

It's the things that we do every day that kill us.

If we had just the occasional drink and cigarette a month our bodies would probably cope. However, twenty a day and a bottle of wine each night will do us in eventually. What if each day we were to do small, positive things to enhance our health instead?

Habits maketh man

Habits make or break us. Twenty years ago I remember looking at a friend of mine and admiring his discipline, tenacity and drive. Twenty years later, he's got it all – a lovely wife, a gorgeously huge home, perfect kids, dogs, and a summer place abroad. He's strong, fit, healthy and, what's more, he's a really nice guy. Don't you just hate him? Habits have made him and have included getting up early, exercising, not smoking or drinking to excess and having a calm mind every single day. We all have mates who have gone down the other road, which was classed as the much cooler road when we were younger. This is the getting trollied road and the doing no exercise road. The trouble is, if you take this road you're likely to wake up at 45 years old, fat, drunk and stupid and that's no way to go through life. You'll pay for that 'animal house' philosophy in the end, however boring it might be in the short term. So what can those of us who overindulge expect?

Smoking gun

The ill effects of smoking take a while to become apparent. To begin with it'll be small things, things that you feel you can cope with because they don't really seem to be doing you any major harm.

Your love life sucks

Smoke smells. Smells linger. Smoke smells linger longer. Clothes, hair, furnishings, cars are all neon signs that say, 'We smoke and we stink but we don't care!' Oddly enough, this is not an attractive prospect to non-smokers, so it cuts down your choice of partners by around 75 per cent.

Smoke and mirrors

Smokers can expect to look old before their time with premature sagging and wrinkles as the habit dries out their skin. Your hair grows thin and loses its bounce and lustre. Your fingers yellow, along with your teeth and you get those delightful hairline wrinkles around your mouth. All classic signs of a smoker.

In the red

Your bank balance will be showing signs of strain as your habit builds up and you begin smoking more and more. Not to mention the higher premiums you'll have to pay for insurance (they expect you to die younger, you see).

Airwaves

Breathing is a brilliant idea. Everybody does it. Your lungs really like it and so does the rest of your body. Strangling yourself is cheaper and a swifter, less painful, option than smoking.

An early sign of lung problems is the well-known smoker's cough. This rapidly becomes a morning ritual, whereby you spend a considerable amount of time coughing up as much accumulated rubbish from your airways as the body can expel. Then there's the cough you seem unable to shake off all winter long. The dry cough is caused by the heat scorching your lungs and air passages. This can sometimes be uncontrollable, taking several minutes to clear.

As time goes on, it's the breathlessness that hits. The stairs become a mountain, small hills are an Everest and you can't run for more than a few yards. Any physical activity leaves you short of breath and your chest hurts if you exert yourself too much.

Heartbeat

Coronary heart disease is nicotine's biggest gift to you. Money may make the world go round but, more importantly, your heart makes your blood go round. No heart, no you. Damage your lungs and you damage your heart. As your smoking cuts down the amount of oxygen absorbed into the blood, so the heart has to work all the harder to pump the necessary amount of oxygen to keep the muscles and vital organs going.

The longer you smoke, the more clogged up the lungs become, the harder the heart has to work. Chest pains are a worrying sign and ought to be a serious warning to you that the heart just can't take it any more.

The problems you'll be causing your blood vessels can lead to a stroke, which can kill you or leave you disabled or unable to speak. Classic warning signs of an impending stroke are double vision, terrible headaches or difficulty finding the right words.

Circulation problems can lead to amputation, particularly of toes, feet and legs. Your teeth will also start to loosen as your smoking causes bone disease and your gums recede.

The only real answer is to stop now. One year after stopping, your risk of having a heart attack falls to about half that of a smoker and within 15 years falls to a level similar to that of a person who has never smoked. Within 15 years of quitting, an ex-smoker's risk of developing lung cancer reduces to only slightly greater than that of a non-smoker.

Sorry guys but I am not convinced this is without side-effects. Emerging research is throwing up all kinds of issues, including that vaping could induce certain cancers and be as bad for your heart as cigarettes. The flavourings are also a concern since they contain a cocktail of chemical compounds.

Secrets of wine

The wine industry might try to promote wine as an intrinsic part of a healthy diet, but there is no doubt that the effects of heavy drinking are calamitous. On an almost weekly basis some new study is published promoting the benefits of wine consumption and is contradicted by another blaming alcohol for a catalogue of ills.

A recent study concluded that even one drink per day is too much. I think we'll find that in time the safe level of alcohol consumption will be dependent on the type of alcohol consumed and the underlying health of the person drinking it. Still, it is probably not a health product.

The grim truth

However much the pro-wine lobby might champion the cause of wine consumption, alcohol is known to be linked to liver and brain damage, cancer, nerve and muscle wasting, blood disorders, raised blood pressure, strokes, skin infections, psoriasis, infertility and birth defects. Alcohol consumption can also be blamed for all sorts of collateral damage such as road accidents and domestic violence. There is no doubt that excessive alcohol consumption has a detrimental effect upon health. If it had been invented in the twentieth century it would almost certainly have been banned. But all studies into health constitute an inexact science. You have to make up your own mind about what you consider safe levels of consumption – and what risks you are prepared to take. What complicates the matter is that alcohol consumption affects us all in different ways. Much depends on our size, gender and metabolism.

Sobering, isn't it?

One fact that undermines the case of the pro-alcohol lobby is that much of the research is sponsored by those who have a vested interest in the continued growth of alcohol consumption. Yet, aside from the rash claims made by studies published by various universities (many of which happen to be located in winemaking regions such as Bordeaux and Burgundy), there is fairly convincing evidence that moderate wine consumption does have some benefits. Drinking moderately, say a glass of wine a day, is believed to reduce the chances of cardiovascular disease, although it is unlikely that it's the alcohol element of the wine that is beneficial – the same benefits could be achieved by drinking grape juice. Despite technically being toxic, alcohol in the form of red wine offers such benefits as controlling the levels of blood cholesterol and blood-clotting proteins.

The problem of cheap alcohol

A growing problem in recent years that is rarely highlighted is the falling price of alcohol; for example, where wine is concerned, the combination of better technology and increased volume of wine being produced has meant that the cost of a bottle has fallen dramatically over the last twenty years. The fact that alcohol is no longer a luxury and so much more accessible has helped to drive up consumption.

One of the great planks of the wine–health debate is based on what is known as the 'French paradox' – the discovery made by US documentary makers that, despite a relatively high intake of alcohol, the French were generally much healthier than people in Anglo-Saxon countries. If this is true, then one of the contributory factors – besides the 'Mediterranean diet' high in fresh fruit and olive oil – might be the rate at which alcohol is consumed. The tendency in many Northern European countries is to binge, i.e. to concentrate drinking into a relatively short period of time. In France, since wine is an intrinsic part of the gastronomic experience, the rule seems to be 'a little but often'.

There is also an argument that those who see drinking as a source of sensual pleasure are likely to drink less wine than those who drink simply to get drunk.

You might find chapters 22, 33 and 77 especially helpful.

5

Work environment getting you down?

Where would you rather work – a dingy, dull office with little natural light, a work station that is crammed into a corner, with an old, clunky keyboard, little contact with colleagues and nowhere to go for a break? Or … imagine your dream office or work location – an open organised office floor plan, overlooking a river, with a properly organised work station, an ergonomic chair, keyboard and screen, a 'chill-out room' for breaks, free workplace 10 minute massage on Fridays … Dream on!

Seriously, there is a proven difference in employee performance depending on how satisfied we are with our work environment – satisfied people give more, work harder for longer and are happier in their work – all for a smallish investment in their work environment.

Anyone who crouches in cramped positions at work will eventually get a bad back. Look at Quasimodo – if he hasn't spent all day, every day hunched over a computer I don't know who has! Take regular breaks or stretch out frequently if you're doing repetitive movements or sitting or standing still for long periods.

When the natural curves of your spine are preserved, there is less compression of your intervertebral discs and less strain on your back ligaments. And it's not just the position of your back you should think of. When all your other joints are well positioned then the strain on your back ligaments and tendons is minimal.

Sitting is the new smoking

Sitting can cause your pelvis to rotate backwards, causing your lumbar spine to bend with it. This then compresses your intervertebral discs and the cartilage between. Raising your arms in front of your body (for instance, typing on a keyboard) or lifting objects while sitting in this position increases the pressure even more. The damage is worse if the muscles around your spine holding you in position become tired.

Being overweight or obese will pull your spine into an unnatural position that makes it more susceptible to wear and tear and may perpetuate your back pain.

A newish trend is for standing desks, or even treadmill desks. We are not designed to sit but to move. Moving all day is key – a couple of frantic sessions in the gym won't compensate for a day of inactivity.

Good employers take their duty of care, enshrined in European Health and Safety legislation seriously. They do workplace assessments before employees get repetitive strain, they encourage people working at PCs to take a ten-minute break every hour and pay for eye tests every year. They go even further … they provide 'healthy working practices' in the form of advice and active guidance and yes, they pay for workplace massages! They conduct job/workplace satisfaction surveys and take regular action in response to feedback. They enable people to personalise their workspaces (within sensible limits), provide real, tended plants and do stress risk assessments to identify sources of excessive pressures at work. They have regular workplace meetings for employees to discuss and resolve concerns about their workplace. Where would you rather work?

You might find chapters 46, 53, 54 and 81 especially helpful.

6
Tiredness and lack of energy

Injury, poor performance and depression – the results of not getting your sleep quota

You're tired during the day, irritable, anxious, have difficulty concentrating and are about as alert as a fridge freezer. If you don't deal with your sleep problem, your health will spiral downwards and your once cheery personality will be replaced by a glum, short-tempered one. Here's what to expect when you're deprived of sleep. It could be worse than you think …

- Poor memory. During a good night's sleep, in the REM stage, the brain busily replenishes the neurotransmitters that organise neural networks vital for remembering, learning, performance and problem solving. If you deprive the brain of sleep, you get less REM sleep. The result? The crossword takes twice as long to finish, you'll forget the names of close friends and you'll stare at the tax form for days before even attempting to fill it out. Research also shows that your brain has a kind of 'night hoover', which clears up damage while you sleep. It's essential that we get enough sleep to allow this work to be done.

- More car accidents. According to one study drowsiness or sleep disorders was a factor in about half of all traffic accidents and 36 per cent of fatal accidents. Another study compared the reaction times between people who were sleep deprived and those who'd been drinking alcohol. The result? Pretty poor mental functioning all round. This suggests that driving when tired is as dangerous as driving drunk

- Constant colds. With a tissue pressed to your face at all times, no one's really seen you properly for weeks – which is probably a good thing considering your dry, flaky red nose, cracked lips and streaming eyes. Recent research demonstrated that the nightly loss of four hours of sleep over ten days in healthy young adults significantly reduced their immune function. The number of white blood cells (responsible for the production of antibodies that fight disease) within the body decreases, as does the activity of the remaining white blood cells.

- Old before your time. Research suggests that missing sleep can actually speed up ageing. Sleeping for only four hours a night for less than a week, reduces the body's ability to process and store carbohydrates and regulate hormone levels – changes which are similar to those of advanced ageing. Another study found that sleeping under five hours per night lowered the lifespan (although sleeping more than nine hours also did the same).

- Makes you fat. Lack of sleep makes you hungry and more prone to putting on weight – one of the main causes of snoring and sleep apnoea. The key to this is the hormone leptin, which signals when the body needs or does not need more food. Leptin levels rise during sleep and this tells your brain that you've eaten enough and don't need any more calories. When you're sleep deprived, leptin levels are low, which sends a signal to your brain that you need more calories. Your brain thinks that there's a shortage of food and that you need to eat more when, in fact, you've eaten enough.

- High blood pressure. Blood pressure usually falls during the sleep cycle; however, interrupted sleep can adversely affect this normal decline, leading to hypertension and cardiovascular problems. One study of nurses showed that those who slept five hours or less had a 45 per cent greater risk of developing heart disease than those sleeping eight hours. Those sleeping nine to eleven hours increased their risk by 38 per cent.

- Diabetes risk. Research has also shown that insufficient sleep impairs the body's ability to use insulin, which can lead to the onset of diabetes.

- Risk of Alzheimers and other degenerative diseases. Research shos that lack of sleep may be a contributory factor. British Prime Minister Margaret Thatcher famously slept for only four hours a night but in later years suffered serious mental decline – could the two have been linked? While the scientists are still working on the links between these diseases and poor sleep it's probably safer to do your utmost to get good quality sleep every night.

You might find chapters 28, 29, 32, 66, 72 and 74 especially helpful.

7

Financial demons

What has money got to do with Wellness? Well messy finances have a way of wreaking havoc on other areas of your life – they're another source of stress and if you're stressed chances are you're not feeling as healthy or happy as you'd like.

Picture the scene. You've been flexing that new credit card far too much. So perhaps you fall behind on your payments. Perhaps you get into a bad habit of spending more than you earned – for the fifth month running. You feel yourself sliding into debt. Your overdraft limit is looming, and you're only halfway through the month. You would try to pay the phone bill but you can't remember where you left it – probably in the same pile as all those receipts/papers for your tax form. Uh-oh.

Your partner gets wind of the credit card gymnastics and isn't happy. The stress starts to take its toll on your health. You borrow more to get back on track, but end up further in debt on credit cards with crippling interest rates. Bailiffs come a-knocking. Partner leaves you for younger, more solvent model. House repossessed. Life in tatters. Die alone surrounded by cats.

See what happens when you don't take your finances by the proverbials? Start by assessing just how organised you are when it comes to income, outgoings – and striking that fine balance. Are you sensibly thinking of the future? Is your pension plan a winner? Do you actually have a pension? Do you invest wisely? Do you actually have a savings plan?

Health experts are bemoaning the fact that we're fast becoming a nation of fatties. The thing about the population carrying a few extra kilos is that it's pretty obvious to the most untrained of eyes. Take a walk down your local high street and watch people waddle. Our readiness to take on previously unheard of levels of debt is a different story. Barring a spectacular fall from monetary grace, our financial health is our secret. How could the couple two doors along afford to have that conservatory built? Who knows? How can the neighbours manage to put all three of their children through private education? How can the office administrator go on quite so many expensive holidays?

What we do know is that collectively we are carrying more on our credit cards and mortgages than any previous generation. The average household has debts of around £53,785 (including what we owe on our mortgages), with many of us owing between six and twelve times our household's annual income. Credit Action reports that 8,465 new debt problems were dealt with by the Citizens' Advice Bureau each working day in the first half of 2012.

Debt's the way to do it

We're debt junkies. Go to college and come out with a qualification and a pile of bills. You've chanced on a bargain in the sales but you're a bit short this month? No problem – stick it on the credit card. Whether it's buying a house or a car or just paying for Christmas, resistance to debt has never been lower.

Somewhere along the line, we've succumbed to the delusion that owing money is sophisticated. We look on that elderly uncle who'll only buy something when there's cash in the bank to pay for it as some kind of financial ingénue rather than as a model of financial prudence.

And, of course, it's getting ever easier to pile up the debt. Credit card companies seem to fall over themselves in their haste to bump up our credit limits, and then send us a letter telling us the 'good news' that our capacity for debt is now that much greater. Damn their eyes.

Used sensibly, credit cards can be a neat budgeting tool, which can provide a bit of financial flexibility. And borrowing money via your credit card can be extremely positive if you use it to buy smartly. Part of the trouble is that most of our credit card spend tends to go on buying liabilities rather than assets. Borrowing money to buy things that go down in value is a very bad habit to develop. Since the 2007 banking crisis we have perhaps become a little more sceptical of financial institutions than we once were.

One other reason not to be in debt is that it prevents us from building up a savings buffer to give us a measure of protection from forces beyond our control, such as future banking crises, Brexit and governmental change.

An average of 314 purchases are made in the UK every second using debit and credit cards, and at the last count the UK's total credit card debt was £55.4 bn. In November 2012 the average interest rate payable on credit card transactions was 18.35% – 17.85% above the Bank of England base rate. Do you know what your total credit card debt is? Do you know what rates of interest you're paying on the cards you use? Chances are they vary quite widely.

So when it comes to getting your finances in check, you need to clarify your objectives. Tick any of the following that apply to you. It may also be worth cutting the list out, or copying it on to a big piece of paper and sticking it on the wall to remind you why you've finally resolved to get more money-organised.

1. I want to be out of debt.

2. I'd like to be able to lay my hands on important bills/receipts/ statements without having to turn the house or office upside down.

3. I'd like to start saving.

4. I'd like to be able to live mortgage-free within the next ten years.

5. I'd like to be more punctual and organised when it comes to paying bills – no more red ones!

6. I need to feel calmer and less flustered when it comes to my finances.

7. I need to start planning for my children's future – university fees, etc.

8. I'd like to overhaul the way I spend my money.

9. I'd like to be able to make more money without doing more work!

10. I'd like to get savvy about the stock market.

11. I'd like to know how to get everything cheaper – give me some bargain-hunter basics.

12. I'd just like to start afresh....

If you ticked four or more, you need a finance-makeover – pronto.

You might find chapter 67 and the box on page 284 especially helpful.

8
Work conditions – bullying and harassment

Bullying exists. Always has done and always will. You'll find bullies everywhere, not just in the classroom and the playground, but also on the building site, in the office and on the shop floor.

Ask any school teacher and most will say that bullying starts at a young age in a minority of children – it is their way of finding their place in the pecking order or getting their way. Unfortunately some children who bullied at school, go on to use those behaviours and tactics in the workplace. However, they learn to be more devious in their bullying, as most organisations do not tolerate overt bullying or the lesser charge of harassment and have policies to deal with such aberrant behaviours.

Our nearest animal relatives – chimpanzees, exhibit extreme bullying behaviours to establish their position in the social hierarchy; the punishment for any ape that challenges the ruling alphas can be very harsh. So it is with humans; it is part of our ancestry and behavioural legacy to put others in their place sometimes, even though our process of socialisation should enable us to find other ways of getting what we want.

So when does a direct and confrontational management style become bullying? Essentially, bullying is in the eye of the beholder – if you feel someone's behaviour is intimidating then it could be viewed as bullying. Wagging a finger in your face, fixing you with a stare and telling you in no uncertain terms that you crossed the line in a meeting by contradicting them – could be viewed as 'strict guidance'. However, if this is part of a pattern of intimidating behaviour used with an individual, then it is likely to be bullying.

Bullying covers a wide range of actions, from name calling, saying or writing hurtful things, leaving colleagues out of activities, not talking to them, threatening them and making them feel scared or making them do things they don't want to do. Some people are more at risk of being bullied, especially those who are deemed somehow different to those around them, jealousy can often be at the root of the problem.

There are various types of bullying:

- Physical; actual or threatened physical violence.

- Verbal, which includes insults, racist, sexist or homophobic comments.

- Psychological – probably the most commonly encountered type of workplace bullying – which covers actions like spreading rumours, excluding and isolating, humiliating or belittling the victim in front of colleagues, giving them too much work so they are bound to fail or be overworked, unfairly passing them over for promotion and blaming them for mistakes or problems that are not their fault.

Bullying can be in person, on the phone or via email and the internet. Most commonly (though not always) the perpetrator is in a more senior position than the person they are bullying.

How should you deal with a bully? Well it takes courage and some guile. The usual recommendation is that you need to 'stand up to a bully' and show that you are not a person to be intimidated, but this is hard if the person doing the bullying is someone in a position of authority. Step 1 – seek confidential advice from another manager or human resource professional. Step 2 – if you feel confident enough – assert yourself with the person concerned, knowing that there is a policy to fall back on. Step 3 – escalate the issue by reporting the situation to someone who can support you. You definitely do not have to put up with it!

Mohandas K. Gandhi said something particularly sage on this subject: 'First they ignore you, then they ridicule you, then they fight you, then you win.' Whether you've been bullied, know someone who is being bullied or are a bully yourself, keep those words in mind. Bullies don't have to win.

According to the Workplace Bullying Helpline 19 million sick days are lost due to bullying per annum. It is not ever the fault of the bullied person and is not a fact of working life that should just be endured. Laws are in place to deal with this kind of behaviour and your organisation should have its own procedures to implement these laws.

You might find chapter 68 and the box on page 276 especially helpful

9
Stress

So you're stressed? Be grateful. Stress makes life a lot sweeter when you learn to manage it right. Better sex, sharper mind, longer life – stress does all this. Which is why so many of us are addicted to it.

Nearly half of people claim to be more stressed today than they were five years ago; over three-quarters of people consider stress as intrinsic to their jobs. But let's look at the positives. Some stress is good. Some stress is necessary. While chronic stress over a period of months is detrimental, feeling a bit 'stressy' once or twice a week could be just the ticket. Here's what that level of stress can do for you.

Stress keeps you young

When you're stressed your adrenal glands produce a hormone called dehydroepiandrosterone – known as DHEA to its friends – which has been shown to keep mice alive longer. It was also noted that the same mice had more luxuriant coats. The hormone is thought to build collagen and elastin (the building bricks of the skin) and this stimulates a younger looking appearance. (The beauty industry has latched onto this and is trying to develop products that contain DHEA. You're ahead of your game, you produce your own.)

Stress makes you smart

DHEA makes your mind sharper. Chronic stress makes you forgetful but short-term stress can make your brain work better for short periods.

Stress lifts your mood

If you're feeling down in the dumps, a bit of stress isn't necessarily terrible. It could be just what you need to perk you up again. Stress forces you to make decisions and take responsibility. Experts believe this protects us from falling into a state of depression. A recent study found that short doses of the stress hormone cortisol protect some people against depression in the way that antidepressants regulate mood. Too much cortisol leads to extreme exhaustion, but just a little bit is fine.

Stress improves your sex life

Let's hear it for our old friend, DHEA. Women with a low libido who were given doses of DHEA got more interested again. It turns out that low levels of stress are linked to control of sex drive. Moderate stress releases DHEA and this affects libido positively.

Stress keeps you alive

A study carried out at the University of Texas showed that people with few pressures are up to 50 per cent more likely to die within ten years of quitting work than those who faced major responsibility. People under regular pressure tend to take better control of their lives and as a result suffer fewer conditions linked to failing finances, poor relationships and employment problems.

Stress works in another way to keep us healthy and alive. Humans are designed to have short, sharp periods of stress every now and then. Stress gives us the 'high' that is necessary for psychological good health. If your life is free of stress you may look to get the highs elsewhere and as result indulge in what psychologists call 'high-risk behaviour.' Translation: extreme sports, dangerous sexual behaviour, fighting, drugs. One way of seeing each of these activities is a way of artificially introducing stress into an understimulated life. Stress keeps us from falling into bad or frankly, mad, habits.

You can't stress-proof your life

Life is innately stressful – we can't completely banish stress from our lives. Even if you lock yourself in your bedroom for the foreseeable future, stress will find you out. Stress is caused by change, and life changes even if you withdraw from it and hide under the bed. The ripples of change will still lap against your bedroom door.

But by learning to manage stress, and use it to your advantage, you can find it motivates, energises and spurs you on to a richer and more fulfilling life. So whenever the pace of life is getting you down remember there's only one thing worse for you than too much stress, and that's too little.

You might find chapters 34, 35, 57 and 59 especially helpful.

10
Burnout

What is burnout? It's when a relationship – either work or personal – has got so bad that you just can't stand it any longer. If the only route of action that appeals is hiding under your duvet until Christmas, it's time to reassess your situation. See how you score on the questions below. Tot up the scores for each statement you agree with.

	Score
You fantasise a lot about your perfect life that doesn't include your dull/annoying partner/job?	+1
You say 'I can't take it any more' at least once a week	+2
You feel unappreciated	+3
Tension is beginning to affect your health	+3
You wake up dreading the day ahead	+3
All you want to do in the evening is slump in front of the TV and sleep	+1

Score

4 or under

Mild level of dissatisfaction. This indicates that the present situation is stressful but potentially saveable.

4–9

Life is not good and you know you need to act.

10 or over

Burnout imminent.

Dr Dina Glouberman, who has written on the subject of burnout, defined it as what happens when 'The love or meaning in what we are doing goes, but attachment drives us to carry on.'

It's this attachment that you need to question. It's clear that some situations are easier to leave than others but if you have tried all you can to fix your particular hell and nothing improves, it's time to admit the unhappiness to yourself and others, and move on. In our competitive world, it's hard to say 'I may have made a mistake.' The more time you've invested in the wrong life, the harder it is to give up on it. But the first step is simply admitting to yourself and perhaps a few trusted compadres that yes, you are human, you made a mistake.

There's nothing wrong with being unhappy with your life. See it as a positive. What it signals is that you have outgrown your present situation and that it's time to move on. Otherwise, the stress of living a life that isn't yours can be fearsome. You risk burnout – a state of collapse where you lose all joy in life. Your body gives out and your spirit gives up. It is extremely painful and can take months, even years to come back from.

But even if you do burn out, it's not an unmitigated catastrophe. For many it's the beginning of a new, more enlightened life. After spending their time in the metaphorical wilderness, they rethink their life and choose a new route.

Here's an exercise to help you get the process started:

- Lie down. Breathe deeply. When you're calm, ask yourself, 'If I woke up and all my problems and worries had gone, how would I know a miracle had happened?'

- How would you behave, talk, walk, think – if the miracle had happened?

- How do you think your family and friends would know a miracle had happened?

- If you were to assess your life right now somewhere between 0 and 10, with 0 being your worst life and 10 a full-scale miracle life, where would this day be on the scale?

- What would need to happen for you to move one step up?

- How would other people know that you had moved one step up?

This exercise helps you realise that it's not so much miracles (externals) that determine your happiness, but your behaviour. You are in control.

You might find chapters 65 and 69 especially helpful.

11
Feeling down, or are you depressed?

All of us feel down sometimes. We may occasionally experience low mood, a lack of motivation, reduced physical energy, and perhaps lowered self-esteem; days when we cannot get our act together or pick ourselves up. When these signs persist over a period of time, then we may be suffering from 'clinical depression'. Depression varies from one person to another in its intensity, persistence and the exact nature of symptoms experienced, but some of the signs are consistent. So if you are consistently experiencing several of the following symptoms then you may be depressed:

- Feeling sad, blue and tearful (low mood, disrupted affect);

- Low physical energy, having trouble getting up in the morning (lethargy);

- Low motivation to tackle problems and take on challenges (apathy);

- Disrupted sleep – trouble getting to sleep, early waking;

- Excessive worrying about your problems, ruminating on issues;

- Excessive self-doubt, reduced self-esteem (low self-worth).

While depression varies in its causes reputable institutes such as the World Health Organization have shown that about 10 per cent of the global population suffers from depression, so you are far from alone – depression appears to be part of the human condition. Certain events and situations make us more prone to developing depression. These include:

- Significant changes in our working lives, e.g. change of role, redundancy, retirement;

- Domestic disruption, e.g. divorce, moving house, debt;

- Mid-life adjustments, e.g. career plateau, children leaving home;

- Grieving for a loved one (bereavement);

- Serious illness, injury or disfigurement;

- Having a baby;

- Menopause or other significant hormonal changes;

- Substance abuse, e.g. alcoholism, drug taking or addiction.

Reactive depression

A proportion of depression is described as 'reactive' (see the first four points, above) – we suffer low mood and associated issues 'in reaction' to something that is happening in our lives that has disrupted our usual emotional balance. We might view this change in mood as helping us adapt or cope by reducing the effort we expend on something that is no longer proving worthwhile. Although in other ways depression is mal-adaptive – just when we need resources and energy to fight a difficult situation or problem, our bodies and brains go into shutdown/ hibernation mode.

Systemic depression

Other forms of depression are more related to physical changes in our bodies; states which disrupt our immune systems, hormonal balance or functioning of our brains (see the last four points, above). For example, seasonal affective disorder (SAD) is a form of depression that occurs in response to a reduction in exposure to sunlight in the winter (hence reducing ultra-violet light and associated vitamin D), which affects some people's moods. This second type of depression could be described as 'systemic' – a state affecting mood or emotion that is partly due to predisposition within the person. Some unfortunate people are more likely to get depression due to their emotional make-up or the way their brain functions. In more extreme forms of depression, such as major depressive disorder, or bipolar disorder, medication or even hospitalisation is required to treat severe symptoms, including suicidal thinking or psychosis.

Treatment for depression

Depression can significantly reduce the quality of our lives. Not only does the condition make us think negatively about ourselves, it affects energy levels, the ability to deal with our problems, and alters our behaviour, e.g. we feel less sociable and confident and avoid challenge and perceived threats. Our self-esteem takes a hit and this affects the choices we make. If we do not think well of ourselves, then that in turn makes it harder for others to think well of us.

Treatment can take the form of medication, i.e. antidepressants, which address the chemical disruptions in our brains associated with being in a depressed state. Antidepressants can help by aiding the 'depressed brain' to recover normal functioning, thereby restoring normal sleep patterns, increasing mood and energy levels.

Recent research has shown that drug treatments may not be the long-term answer in over 50 per cent of depression cases and that using techniques to change our thinking about ourselves should be a vital part of the treatment for depression. The underlying assumption is that we contribute to our own depression by unhealthy ways of thinking about ourselves, such as, 'I am not good enough – I always mess up friendships'.

The treatment most commonly used is known as Cognitive Behavioural Therapy (CBT) and aims to adopt an 'active problem-solving approach' to tackling the causes and impacts of depression, initially with the support of a counsellor or therapist. For instance, getting a depressed person to list all the positive contributions they have made to other people's lives, or encouraging them to give time to charitable causes or people in need. Appreciating positive contributions is an antidote to the feelings of low self-worth, commonly associated with depression. CBT encourages depressed people to become aware of their thoughts about themselves and to challenge negative thoughts, replacing them with positive ones.

Work it out

Many people feel like walking out of jobs when they're depressed. You may have good reasons for hating work, but a better course of action would be to concentrate on getting better; put off making major decisions like resigning until you are. When you're depressed, you've probably got a low opinion of yourself, which means it's much harder to write applications and shine at interviews, preventing you from getting the sort of work you deserve. If you feel factors at work are making your depression worse, talking this through with occupational health or your own doctor can be much more helpful than walking out.

If work pressures do start to get you down tell a trusted senior colleague you're feeling under par. They might be able to take some of the pressure off. Many people who are depressed, find it hard to concentrate on written work, but can do mechanical or routine tasks. If there are any physical jobs you could do instead of heavy-duty brain work, get stuck in. Try to avoid hiding at your desk during the lunch break. Whether you like to chill out by the water cooler or cosy up with a cappuccino, chat to colleagues during breaks.

With depression, it is important not to suffer in silence or seek refuge in alcohol or other drugs (which can worsen symptoms). There are positive therapies – medication, counselling or CBT, which can really make a difference. The sooner you get support, the sooner you will restore your emotions to their normal healthy balance.

You might find chapters 36, 62, 74 and 79 especially helpful.

12
Relationship woes

The number of couples divorcing worldwide is increasing year after year. In many countries, more than half of couples who've said 'I do' are now saying 'I don't'. In the UK the number of divorces per year is almost half the number of marriages.

So, should we start issuing divorce papers with every marriage certificate to save time? Well not every country is reporting a race towards marital meltdown. Italy reports only 12 per cent of marriages ending in divorce, Cyprus 13 per cent, Spain 17 per cent and Greece 18 per cent. Maybe it's the Mediterranean climate or something they put in the olive oil, but marriages in these sunny climes are far more likely to last the course than those in many other countries.

What makes the difference? Why is divorce an epidemic in some countries and a rare disease in others? Will geography determine the success of your marriage, or are there any preventive measures, short of moving to Tuscany, that you can take?

In a relationship, life is apt to take over and we can begin to drift apart without realising that it's happening. Suddenly we can find that we don't actually know each other any more. Setting aside time to develop a relationship, no matter how long we've been in it, is one of the most important things that we can do if we value this partnership as a lifelong commitment.

Where is the problem?

Let's look at a work situation first. There are two types of work activities: maintenance and development. Maintenance activities cover things that you do on a daily basis just to get your job done and include selling, taking orders, answering the phone, opening the mail, etc. Development activities are different in that they are one-off tasks and may include designing a new product, launching a new computer system, reorganising the office so that it operates more smoothly, and so on. Maintenance activities are things that we measure (have we reached our sales target?), are highly visible (we haven't and everybody sees the figures), affect the here and now (how are we going to pay the salaries this month?) and are low risk. Development activities, on the other hand, are the complete opposite. So, not surprisingly, everyone is drawn towards maintenance activities. Yet an organisation that doesn't invest time in development activities is liable to be overtaken quickly by its competitors and go bust.

A relationship is the same. When we first fall in love it's all about development activities – getting to know each other, exploring each other's hobbies, finding new hobbies that you could do together, and so much more. Then we move in together and perhaps get married. And what takes over? Maintenance activities like cleaning the house, working all hours to pay the mortgage, shopping and cooking. And then children come along and the problem escalates! The cost of living rises, we become full-time chauffeurs and household chores double. And what now happens to the time that we used to spend together developing our relationship and getting to know each other even better? That comes somewhere near the bottom of our priorities.

How often do you find yourself writing in a Christmas card, 'We really must get together this year'? Worse, you then find yourself writing the same thing in next year's card. So, now think about how important your special relationship is. Does it deserve the time to continually develop so that you can become closer and closer?

You might find chapters 66, 69 and 70 especially helpful.

Part 2
Eating for Wellness

13
What goes in must come out

We all know that what goes in at the top comes out in a different form at the bottom. But what happens in between? And why is it so important that all the different components of the digestive system are working properly?

It all starts when you first smell that delicious roast chicken your mum is cooking for dinner. As the aroma wafts up the stairs and into your room and your nostrils, powerful chemical messages are set in motion to get us ready to digest and assimilate food. Chewing food is particularly important in getting enzymes, which break down food, ready for work as the food is passed into the stomach, which acts like a soft-walled concrete mixer. Except, of course, that you're actually churning food in a man-made soup of hydrochloric acid. Far from being a bad thing, this stomach acid is crucial, and poor digestion may be down to not having enough of this acid. If you're worried about not having enough, try relaxing at meal times (stress shuts down your digestive system) or get a qualified nutritionist to test your stomach acidity and recommend how to improve your digestive health. There's some controversy about drinking with meals and some experts are actually convinced that liquid waters down your digestive fire, making it less effective. If, like most people, you're worried about having too much stomach acid (reflux, acid burn), check out your lifestyle and diet (drinking too much?) or think about being tested for food intolerances.

Gut feeling

Once your stomach has finished all that churning, your food is passed to the next bit of the processing machine, your small intestine, which is anything but small. Your food is digested and absorbed here so that you can function. One of the most important organs that helps do all this clever stuff is the pancreas, which neutralises the acid mixture that leaves the stomach and then secretes specific chemicals or enzymes to break down the food into smaller particles.

If you feel that your digestion isn't quite what it should be, why not try food combining? There are massive tomes on this, such as *The Food Combining Bible* by Jan Dries and Inge Dries, but put at its simplest it means eating carbohydrates and proteins at separate meals but never together. You must also eat fruit away from other food. Sir John Mills was a huge fan of this way of eating for much of his long life. Food combiners say that it does wonders for the digestion, as all the different enzymes aren't competing against each other.

Liver little longer

It's your liver – a wonder of engineering – that gets the hardest time of all. It helps to emulsify fats and it breaks down hormones, including cholesterol. Your liver manufactures 13,000 chemicals and has 2,000 enzyme systems! You've got to keep it in top nick or you'll start to feel a bit off-colour. I hate to spoil your fun, but drinking is obviously the big baddy in terms of making the liver work harder than it should.

The liver produces fluid called bile, which is stored in the gall bladder. When we eat, the gall bladder and liver release bile into the duct that connects the liver, gall bladder and pancreas to the small intestine. Bile helps emulsify fats, making it easier for them to be digested. An easy supplement to add into your diet is lecithin, which helps your body to emulsify fat. You can even get it from some supermarkets, and your local health-food store should also oblige.

Nearly there...

The last bit of digestion is when what's left of your grub – by this time mainly water, bacteria and fibre – enters the large intestine. About 12 litres (2.5 gallons) of water pass through the large intestine daily, two-thirds from body fluids alone. The large intestine is where your friendly bacteria live. It's quite a teaming life-centre in there! Friendly bacteria are sensitive little souls, so look after them well by not getting too stressed and by eating foods that nurture them, like vegetables. They love fibre. You have a responsibility now! Trillions of little lives are depending on you. Apparently, they're so sensitive that they can even be killed off by loud rock music. In recent years gut environment and contents have risen in our consciousness. We are starting to realise the importance of our 'microbiome', the effect on immune-system health and the connection with the brain. So, take care of your mini ecopark. In fact, why not increase the friendly bacteria in your gut by getting a good acidophilus supplement, or better still by eating more of the foods your gut bacteria will thrive on, such as kefir and sauerkraut?

We all know what happens next. The large intestine is connected to the anus, where the end product of digestion is excreted. This gives rise to all sorts of jokes and is a particular obsession with the British. In other parts of Europe, examining this end product is seen as a good way to diagnose your internal health. Those German toilet bowls with the handy internal shelf are built like that for a reason. For example, a pale, floating stool could mean you're not digesting fat properly and you could amend your diet to take this into consideration. One way to improve this process is to increase the fibre in your diet by upping the amount of vegetables and fruit that you consume. And don't forget to increase the amount of water you're drinking too. If absolutely nothing is happening in this department or your bowels are very slow, consider supplementing fibre in the diet. Psyllium husk is a good way to do this and is available from health shops.

14
Digestion up close and personal

An inefficient bowel is the genesis of several major degenerative diseases, including cancer. Good health starts with good digestion, so let's take a closer look at yours.

Your bowels need to be working very efficiently in order to remove the body's waste. They reabsorb water to be recycled by the body and without an efficient digestive system the result will be like a washing machine where the wastepipe feeds straight back into the drum.

The beet goes on

Which brings us to my favourite topic: stools. An important measure of bowel performance is transit time – how long it takes from the time you eat a food until it comes out the other end. The most effective way to measure this is to eat three or four whole beetroots. This is because beetroot can turn the stool bright red and so if you take note of when you eat the beets you can calculate how long your own personal transit time is. Twelve to 24 hours is the optimal transit time. Sweetcorn works well too – you should spot recognisable corn emerging out the other end. If it's less than 12 hours it's possible that you're not absorbing all the nutrients you should be from your food. More than 24 hours indicates that the wastes are sitting inside your bowel for too long and this can greatly increase the risk of colon disease.

If you've done this experiment and found that your transit time is slow, you'll be relieved to hear that all isn't lost.

One of the major elements in your diet to increase is fibre, and generally you can do this pretty easily by upping the amount of vegetables, fruit and pulses (e.g. lentils) you're eating. Whole grains are also full of fibre, so adding these to your diet will help too. By whole grains I mean unprocessed grains, because processing removes all of the husk and the fibre, which is why brown rice is so much better for you than white. A word of warning though: because of the healthy associations attached to brown bread, some processed loaves are coloured to give them a healthy colour. Look for the key phrase 'wholemeal' to avoid this particular trick. Bread should be heavy and more brick-like – light and fluffy says a lot of air and not much substance. Some experts are saying that while you can keep piling on the vegetables you should be careful not to eat too many grains.

Increasing your water intake is vital. Water shortages do for your digestion pretty much what they do for any other living thing.

Foods that react negatively in the gut include sugar, alcohol, high-fat foods and junk foods like chips and pastries, to name but a few of the major culprits. Foods made up of flour are particularly able to slow everything down in there. Remember making glue from flour and water when you were at school? The same principle applies here.

Friend or foe?

Your insides are prime real estate. You have between about 400 and 500 different bacteria living in your bowels. A total of one hundred trillion bacteria live in your entire digestive system comprising a total weight of about four pounds, and the majority of these guys live in your colon. Some kinds of bacteria are goodies, some are baddies and some don't affect our health at all. The trick is not to let the baddies overwhelm our system and cause an imbalance leading to ill health.

The goodies aren't just in there for the ride, they actually have a major effect on our good health. These guys manufacture many vitamins, including from the important B group, and make some minerals more bioavailable. They also help increase our resistance to food poisoning and are a vital part of our immune system. They can even work to prevent tumours and cancers. To get more of these desirable tenants into your system, eat more cultured foods like yoghurt, sauerkraut and cottage cheese. There are also a number of yoghurts now available containing 'live bacteria' (such as bifidus). If yoghurt leaves you cold, you could take a friendly bacteria supplement. Just one tablet can represent the equivalent of fifteen small tubs of yoghurt, which would take a long time to get through using the traditional teaspoon technique! Your first line of defence however should be a change in diet. Popping pills may well not be necessary and should only be done once this avenue has been explored.

15
Vital energy

Have you ever felt like curling up under your desk and spending the afternoon snoozing? Or been in serious need of matchsticks to prop your eyelids open? And do you ever wonder why this always seems to happen in the middle of a vital meeting, despite three cups of coffee?

The energy equation

We need sugar (glucose) to fire our system. It's the fuel that gives us our energy. However, too much is deemed by our body to be dangerous (think of diabetics).

We obtain this fuel largely from our food. A hormone called insulin specifically lowers these blood sugar levels and adjusts them according to our minute-by-minute needs. We don't have very much sugar circulating at any one time because as soon as we do, in comes insulin to normalise the level. When blood sugar levels are low, we rely on stored glucose (glycogen) found in the muscles and the liver, which helps maintain this delicate equilibrium. Once stored glucose is used, more food will be required to sustain glucose production.

Not all food was created equal. Some foods 'burn' (meaning they're converted into sugar) quickly while other foods 'burn' slowly. These foods are called low and high glycaemic index foods (GI foods). The GI index is a way of measuring foods that are converted to glucose at different rates. You may also have heard mention of a much more complex index called the Glycaemic Load (GL) but for our purposes the GI is adequate. But don't get hung up on the GI index, as confusingly you'll see it published in different places with different values. As a very simple rule of thumb, white things (e.g. potatoes, pasta, bread, parsnips, white rice) are like rocket fuel while dense, thick, fibrous, brown or green things (e.g. lentils, chickpeas, broccoli and other whole, unprocessed foods) are going to burn more slowly and are our great energy sustainers. For example, whereas glucose (sugar) scores 100 on the GI scale, a lentil comes in at a cool 42. The important thing to remember is that it isn't necessarily foods that we traditionally think of as sweet that cause the problems. A 'sweet' potato, for instance, actually scores quite low, as it is wonderfully fibrous.

You can raise your blood sugar by another mechanism. Stick your head in the mouth of a man-eating shark, then quickly take it out again and swim like hell for the shore. This would certainly pick your blood sugar up rapidly, as powerful stress hormones would raise blood sugar to give you enough energy for your clever exit strategy. We do this all the time, but usually our boss, gas bill or deadline is the cause of our stress and not man-eating sharks. Of course there is an easier way of picking up blood sugar levels – have a fag or a cup of coffee. These are both stimulants, which stimulate the adrenal glands (where those stress hormones come from) to release sugar from storage. But what goes up, must come down, hence staying awake in the meeting becomes a challenge.

So, what's the problem with the blood sugar whizzing up and down all the time? First, the pancreas, where all that insulin is produced is going to get worn out. Second, you're going to get dips of energy as the blood sugar levels plummet when insulin tries to lower them. Third, insulin is also a fat storage hormone, so if it overreacts and there's continuously too much insulin in the system, eventually you'll put on weight. Commonly this appears as those cute love handles or that attractive tyre round the middle. And where do you see this phenomenon most commonly? On executives who are eating the wrong things, having too many cups of coffee and getting stressed out.

There is no easy solution. There is no such thing as healthy convenience food. To eat well for blood-sugar balance you by and large have to eat what I call *real* food, in other words unprocessed wholefoods.

If you don't have the time to go shopping try shopping online. Once it's set up it's wonderfully easy. Ones that promise hour delivery slots are best, otherwise you have to hang around for them to deliver, which is a pain. The key phrase is, 'Be prepared.'

All about blood sugar

Your body can only deal with one to two teaspoons of sugar in the blood at any one time. So, if, for example, you drank a bottle of a glucose-based sports drink – the sugar in the blood would rise steeply. The body protects itself from too much sugar in the blood by releasing a hormone called insulin. Insulin lowers the sugar in the blood rapidly. It is a fat storage hormone – unfortunately if there is too much insulin released it will encourage the storage of the foods you eat as fat. Therefore you need to keep your levels of blood sugar stable in order to prevent the release of too much insulin so that you can reduce fat storage and lose weight, and in order to maintain a steady flow of energy.

I have devised a very easy way to follow a lower glycaemic index system without having to count or know what each individual food scores. How quickly a food releases its sugar is measured on a scale called Glycaemic Index. Sweet, fluffy and white foods (e.g. ripe bananas, white bread, cake) have a high GI score and cause blood sugar to rise rapidly. Thick (dense), fibrous, protein foods (e.g. oats, rye, pulses, eggs) have a low GI score and do not release their sugars rapidly, keeping blood sugar more stable.

Slow burn foods are:

Thick (dense), fibrous, protein = low GL

Fast burn foods are:

Sweet, fluffy and white = high GL

Adding fibre and protein makes food burn more slowly. For example, if you had an apple and you ate it with a handful of nuts it would burn more slowly. Or if you had a sweet potato and added some fish it too would burn more slowly.

Keeping your blood sugar more stable helps maintain energy; it prevents the mid-afternoon slump, helps maintain a healthy weight and also keeps stress under control because the blood sugar is not swinging around. Stable blood sugar also helps keep cravings under control – e.g. cravings for sugar, alcohol or caffeine – as these act as stimulants to prop the blood sugar up.

16
Sugar bites back

I can understand why the public at large is wholly confused by nutrition and all its messages. One minute you should drink red wine for health, the next the advised alcohol units are reduced by the government advisory folk.

For the last thirty years we've all been told to avoid saturated fats but then butter makes a comeback (and isn't butter a saturated fat?). During those thirty years when we've been told to avoid saturated fat, the world's collective waistline has continued expanding at ever more alarming rates. So if we are avoiding dietary fat, what is it that is making us 'fat, sick and nearly dead'?*

It starts with a love affair, one that began innocently enough. But like the tragic tale of Romeo and Juliet, it's such a passionate compulsion that this love addiction has resulted in death and destruction. Yes, our love affair with sugar has not only cost the earth (in terms of an environmental impact) but it could actually be killing us too.

From our very first mouthful of breast milk, which is naturally sweet, we are compelled to feed ourselves with sweetness. In nature, food that is poisonous is not generally sweet, and sweet foods are hard to come by, so our instinct pulls us towards luscious sweetness. It feels safe, nurturing, and indulgent. But

---

* I take this phrase from Joe Cross's biographical documentary of the same name, which is well worth watching.

since the sixteenth century we have seen a massive rise in the amount of sugar in our diet, and it's having a cost. In earlier centuries the human cost was paid by the slaves forced to work on plantations but these days it is making all of us sick. Is sugar biting us back?

It's thought that sugar was used in the Polynesian Islands over 5,000 years ago. Winding forward, it seems that in 510 BC Darius, the Persian Emperor, arrived in the Indian subcontinent to find that people were sweetening their food with sugar cane – up until that point, the Persians had used honey. They gave this 'new' plant the rather catchy title of 'the reed which gives honey without bees'. By the fourth century, Alexander the Great was referring to sugar cane as 'the sacred reed', and its black-magic influence had spread to Greece and Rome. The Arabs who invaded Persia in the seventh century became enamoured of the sugar-cane plant, and introduced all sorts of places to sugar, including Egypt, Rhodes, Cyprus, North Africa, Southern Spain and Syria. They took sugar to Spain and Portugal, and from there Christopher Columbus took the plant to the Caribbean island of Santa Domingo in 1493, where the plant flourished.

In the Americas, the Jamestown colony was established by 1609 and by 1619 sugar and slaves were present. Sugar was to become so profitable that it was known as 'white gold'. Thirty thousand tonnes of sugar were being produced by 1750 but it was taxed heavily and it wasn't until until 1874 when the British parliament abolished the sugar duty that it became more affordable to ordinary people. By this time, the natural environments of the Caribbean were wrecked, huge numbers of people were enslaved, displaced and dehumanised – all in the pursuit of an addictive white powder – sugar.

The eighteenth century's love of tea and coffee sweetened with sugar elevated this treat food into an everyday commodity. Gradually, sugar trickled down to the working classes in the nineteenth century as cheap, sugary jam became a mainstay of the diet. Per capita sugar consumption went from 4 lbs in 1704 to 90 lbs in 1901. Tea was the drum-banging message of the temperance movement – the poor were encouraged to move off alcohol and into sugary tea. Ironically weak beer had nutritional value, while the tea actually leached valuable nutrients, and the sugar didn't help. It's hard to believe, but when they were first introduced coke and other carbonated drinks were considered the healthy choices. And so our love affair with sugar has continued to the modern day with convenience food stacked full of sugar. This sector has grown by seventy per cent in the last ten years, so we now spend a third of our total food budget on convenience foods. Government is a willing partner in promoting British food interests – we are very good at manufacturing junk food, and the sugar lobby is an active one.

Where did it all go wrong?

According to the World Health Organization, rates of obesity doubled between 1980 and 2014. 'Professor Sugar', Robert Lustig, makes a convincing case for our consumption of sugar lying at the root of this explosion.* Interestingly, it is not only fat people getting sick, it's potentially all of us. It is tempting to look at the fat people and blame them for their condition but with the food industry adding sugar and other undesirable ingredients to our food – often under pseudonyms, we can be totally unaware what exactly is in our food.

Back in 1972 British scientist John Yudkin argued in his book *Pure, White and Deadly* – that sugar was the big issue, but American Ancel Keys convinced the world it was fat that was responsible for poor health. It now seems that a study which appeared to show that high fat diets caused heart attacks, was (shall we say) doctored to leave out inconvenient evidence suggesting that fat

---

*   His take on sugar and the cause of our expanding waistline and decline in health is worth watching in full: www.youtube.com/watch?v=dBnniua6-oM.

didn't cause heart disease. Needless to say, Yudkin and his alarm about sugar was ignored (at best) and discredited (at worst) by an industry with a bottom line to take care of.

While table sugar is a problem, the issue says Lustig is fructose (a type of simple sugar), added to junk food, especially to fizzy drinks. The conventional argument is that a calorie is a calorie and it doesn't matter if you are eating 100 calories of broccoli or 100 calories of candy, they will still be 100 calories. Unfortunately, our bodies are more complicated than that – we are not a closed system like a boiler, or Stephenson's *Rocket*. Our bodies process different foods in different ways. Fructose is processed like alcohol and can contribute to non-alcoholic fatty liver disease for example. So when you give your children fruit juices (which are naturally high in fructose) you give them a substance that in effect can potentially cause the same damage to the liver as alcohol.

There are even differences in the way the body handles different types of sugar. For example, although glucose and fructose seem very similar, glucose can be metabolised efficiently by the body's cells but fructose must be processed by the liver to be stored as fat. Fructose doesn't shut off the body's hunger hormone (ghrelin) like glucose does so you eat more when you eat fructose.

Something called the thermic effect means that what type of food a calorie comes from determines how it is 'burned' by the body. Some food will take more effort to burn than others – protein takes more energy to process than carbohydrates – which is why, gram for gram, some foods make you feel fuller than others.

So what is wrong with a bit of sugar then?

We love sugar but (sob, weep and gnashing of teeth) sugar doesn't love us back. Here are just a few reasons:

1. Sugar is a source of empty energy – it doesn't give us any worthwhile nutrients, so when we consume it all we are getting is simple calorific energy.

2. Fructose sugar processes in a similar way to alcohol.

3. Sugar is inflammatory. It causes spikes in insulin (a hormone that controls sugar in the blood), and when insulin is spiking it can damage tissue and blood vessels. There is a big body of thought that says that inflammation is at the root of all degenerative disease.

4. In addition to messing with our blood sugar (our energy management), there is an argument that says that sugar is chemically addictive.

5. Consuming too much sugar is ageing since consumption of sugar causes oxidation (rusting).

So it would seem that the best course of action is to break-up with sugar and never look back. It's tricky though because sugar is everywhere – in everything processed, from a yoghurt to a savoury sauce, some of which have as many as 6.5 teaspoons of sugar per serving. Not what you were expecting.

You can begin by cutting out the obvious sugar hits:

1. Office cake run. Office birthdays can be perilous for the sugar-conscious individual, but just take a little to be polite, and then bin it when nobody's looking.

2. Eat fruit in its full and natural form (as fruit) and don't drink it as juice – the fibre in the fruit will help slow down the processing of sugar so your blood sugar level doesn't spike. Try not to overdo the amount of fruit in your diet and instead increase the quantity of vegetables you eat.

3. Avoid low-fat processed food – it's usually stuffed with sugar to compensate for the fact that removing all that fat makes it taste horrible.

4. Read your labels carefully and learn the names manufacturers hide sugar behind. Even better don't eat food with labels on it – eat real food.

5. Avoid artificial sweeteners – that is a whole other story. The body finds it difficult to process man-made chemicals and the long-term outcome on our health is uncertain.

6. Learn to drink your tea without sugar and ditch the sugary fizzy drinks.

7. Avoid all those free sugars – including syrups, sugar, honey, fruit concentrates – that are added to food. Just eat real (i.e. unprocessed) food. Yes, I am repeating myself!

In short, sugar has bitten back in terms of:

- The human cost – slavery and ongoing poor working conditions in the sugar industry.

- Ecological impact – destruction of rainforest and other natural habitats to make way for sugar plantations, and the energy required to extract sugar.

- Health cost – a ticking time bomb with your health, and more to the point your children's health. Sugar is everywhere – start with that awareness.

The good news is that now you're aware of the issues you can start protecting your health and that of your family. If we all reduce our sugar consumption we'll be helping the environment too.

17
Nutrition: the basics

There are so many different diets and ways of eating that it's no wonder we're thoroughly confused. Eating for energy by controlling your blood sugar (see page 73) is probably best for handling stress and fuelling Wellness at work but, to begin with, here are some general nutritional guidelines.

One minute vitamin C is good for you, the next it's causing cancer. We all change to margarine, then lo and behold we're told to change back to butter. Let's try to make sense of it all.

The food we eat can be divided up into three major 'macro' nutrient groups: carbohydrates, proteins and fats.

Curb the carbs?

The body uses carbohydrates (carbs) as its main fuel. Carbs can be divided into two types: 'fast burning' (junk food, processed food, honey, sweet foods) and 'slow burning' (whole grains, fresh fruit and veg, grains). The type of carbs you should curb are the fast-burning carbs because these will give you a surge of energy followed by a nasty crash. And avoid rocket-fuel carbohydrates such as white bread, white rice, cakes, biscuits and sugar. Complex carbohydrates usually have more fibre in them to slow down the way sugar is released into your system.

Perfect protein

Protein contains the building blocks (amino acids) that are used for making enzymes, hormones, antibodies and neurotransmitters as well as for repair of the body and for growth. Protein isn't just about huge slabs of juicy steak. Vegetarian sources of protein are important to consider and include beans, tofu, quinoa (a type of seed) and lentils. Aim to eat plenty of vegetarian sources, which are less acid forming, and also consider some cheese and eggs, but not in excess. If you eat meat, have it no more than three times a week.

Fear of fat

A fear of fat has been drummed into us but recently fat has crept back into favour – as long as it is the right type of fat. There are two main types of fat: saturated fats (hard fat) and unsaturated fats. There are also two main categories of unsaturated fats: monounsaturated (olive oil is in this group) and polyunsaturated. Some polyunsaturated fats are good for your brain and generally make the body work efficiently. In fact, they're known as essential fatty acids (EFAs) – the name speaks for itself. EFAs are destroyed by heat and light so, despite some manufacturers' health claims, the benefits of these fats are likely to have been destroyed once foods are processed. Each day, supplement a pure fish oil, eat a good handful of nuts and seeds and avoid the type of fats found in processed foods.

18
What's in what?

Which foods should you target for well-being? Here's a quick guide to what's in your food.

The key to a great diet is variety. This will ensure that you get a broad spectrum of nutrients – vitamins and minerals for everyday health.

A nutritional rainbow

The rule of thumb is to eat as many different coloured foods as possible throughout the day. Coloured food is full of nutrients – look for reds, greens, yellows, oranges and all the colours in between. These will give you antioxidant vitamins that can protect you from disease. A broad spectrum of vitamins and minerals is really important.

I'm not going to go through every vitamin and mineral here, but I'd like to highlight the B group of vitamins, which are very important to our nervous system. They're found in a wide array of foods, but particularly in grains. I'd also like to highlight vitamin C, which is found in berries, citrus fruits, tomatoes and potatoes. Of the minerals, a key one to top up on is calcium, which is found in almonds, sesame seeds and vegetables (that's where cows get their calcium from to provide calcium-rich milk). Among other things, we need calcium for bone and teeth formation, as well as nerve and muscle function. Zinc is another top mineral as it's essential to most bodily functions, including fertility and brain function. Zinc is found in shellfish, lentils, pumpkin seeds and eggs. Before we leave this lightning tour of vitamins and minerals I'd like to mention selenium, another mineral worthy of top billing. Selenium is another antioxidant and it may help prevent cancer. It's naturally found in wheatgerm, tomatoes, onions, broccoli, garlic, eggs, liver and seafood. If you want to know more about vitamins and minerals and where to find them, a great book worth investing in is *The Optimum Nutrition Bible* by Patrick Holford. A classic book on nutrition, it is also informative and easy to read.

So, why do we need vitamins? Well, they're essential to life. They contribute to good health by assisting the biochemical mechanisms in the body and help metabolism. They're considered micronutrients, as the body needs them in tiny amounts to make everything run smoothly. Vitamins work with enzymes to make functions work in the body. There are two main categories: water-soluble vitamins, which must be taken into the body daily, and oil-based vitamins, which can be stored (these include vitamins, A, C, E and K). Minerals come in different forms. The major minerals, such as calcium, magnesium and potassium, form part of the structure of bones and organs. These are needed either in high milligrams or even gram quantities on a daily basis. Then there are the trace elements, which are important for biochemical reactions in the body. Become deficient in any of these and eventually some part of your body will begin to grind to a halt.

Variation in the diet is the key to expanding the possibility of a wide choice of vitamins and minerals. Due to modern methods of transporting and storing food, even the freshest food can be nutrient deficient. Mineral levels in food are decreasing at an alarming rate because modern farming methods are depleting the soil of nutrients. You may wish to supplement your diet with a good multivitamin and mineral supplement. A qualified nutritionist will help you make a good choice.

The mythical 'balanced diet' is difficult to define, so how do you know if you personally are getting one? Variety is the spice of life. Eat all sorts of different coloured vegetables, grains and fruit, different kinds of oily fish and, if you eat meat, organic, grass-fed meat occasionally. Because of our mineral-depleted crops, in the West we're not malnourished in terms of calories but we are malnourished in terms of nutrients. There might be some merit in choosing a good multivitamin. However, remember that most supplements are produced chemically.

19
Get organic

With more and more headlines screaming at us every day about unsafe food, is it any wonder that we're turning to organic food in our droves? But is it worth it?

From pesticide residue in pears to mercury poisoning from tuna, it's no wonder we're unsure about what's safe. But aside from this, we're turning to organic because of the taste. Remember how tomatoes should taste? Quite simply, like organic ones.

Production means prizes

Farmers have been under a huge amount of pressure to increase productivity, but at a cost. Many non-organic fruit and vegetables contain a wide range of weedkillers, pesticides and fertilisers to increase food production. Fruit and vegetables also have to look perfect for supermarkets to accept them. Gnarled or pitted products are simply not accepted. But what effects do these chemicals have on human health?

It seems that we know that pesticide residues can cause anxiety, hyperactivity, digestive problems and muscle weakness. Children are particularly vulnerable, as their immune systems aren't fully up and running and their comparatively small body mass means that chemicals are more concentrated.

And it's not just fruit and vegetables that we have to worry about. The biggest risks and the biggest worries come in the form of meat products: crazy cows, potty pigs – it's no joke. The many years of intensive farming in crowded conditions has reaped a whole host of health concerns. It's just not possible to crowd animals into such tight spaces without using industrial strength chemical agents to get rid of the threat of spreading disease.

Feeding on demand

We're so used to having exotic fruit and vegetables out of season and on demand that at first it's difficult to accept that we can only get organic fruit and vegetables that are in season. Of course, a lot of organic food is produced abroad and flown to our supermarkets and this makes it more available, but vitamin and mineral content is depleted if food has been on a long journey, and what is the environmental cost? It's therefore much better to buy locally produced products if you can. Many supermarkets are cottoning on to the fact that organic means big business. But remember that just because it says its organic on the packet, it doesn't mean that it's better for you, especially if it has been processed. Once organic products have been turned into a crisp, cake or biscuit, for example, you'll have more or less the same concerns attached to the conventional versions of these foods: high sugar and fat.

So don't be had!

Expect the inspection

The term 'organic' is defined in law and can only be used by farmers who have an organic licence. These farmers have to follow guidelines on how to produce food to organic standards and they're inspected regularly to make sure that these standards are being met. Visit the Soil Association's web site to discover the ins and outs of organic certification in the UK.

Do I buy organic foods? Yes, and I think it's worth it. I always make sure that any meat, eggs or fish is organic and I get organic fruit and vegetables when they're available. I have a box delivered to my door. You'll probably find details of an organic home delivery company at your local health-food shop. I'm now very aware of what fruit and vegetables are in season. And instead of looking in a recipe book and going out to buy what I need, I simply look in the box and create my menus around what I'm given.

Another solution is to prioritise. The government advises that carrots, apples and pears should be peeled as they absorb insecticides through the skin, which could make them unsafe. Buying organic could be a better option. Conventionally farmed salmon are treated with pesticides to prevent mite infestations and there are fears that the chemicals become concentrated in the fish. And choose organic milk and beef, as 'normal' cows are, in some countries, treated with hormones and other growth promoters.

If you can't afford to buy organic, add a generous splash of vinegar to the water when you're giving your vegetables a scrub. There are also products, such as Veggi Wash, that claim to remove pesticides from your fruit and vegetables.

20
Superfoods

What exactly are superfoods? Hero carrots with a mission to save the world?

In their own small way superfoods are indeed our own personal superheroes, as they're foods that have beneficial effects on our health.

Often the best way to get the best from these superfoods is to juice them so that their goodness is easy to absorb. Let's run through a few of the top superfoods which you could incorporate into your juicing repertoire. Well, 'a' is for apple and unsurprisingly apples are a number one superfood. In fact, the well-known herbalist Maurice Messegue once said, 'If you could plant only one tree in your garden, it should be an apple tree.' So, now you know. Apples contain plenty of vitamin C, and the pectin in apples helps keep cholesterol levels stable. Pectin also protects us from pollution. On top of all this, the malic and tartaric acid in apples help neutralise the acid by-products of indigestion and help your body cope with dietary excesses.

Beetroot was used in Romany medicine as a blood-builder for patients who looked pale and run down. Don't overdo it though, as beetroot is such a powerful detoxicant that too much could be a strain on your system. Broccoli is another big superhero. It has been demonstrated in a number of studies to have a protective effect against cancer. And yet another superfood is the humble carrot. Carrots are so rich in betacarotene that a single carrot will supply a whole day's worth of vitamin A requirements. Carrots are also a number one cancer protector.

A great ingredient to add into a juice is a little bit of ginger. Ginger is anti-inflammatory, helps colds, flu and chest congestion, and has been used for centuries as a remedy against sickness and nausea. Another great additive to a juice is parsley, which is full of vitamins A and C and bursting with manganese, iron, copper, calcium, phosphorous, sodium, potassium and magnesium. It acts as a blood purifier.

Although I've picked out just a few here, most fruit and vegetables are of course superfoods. Each and every one has some benefit to our health. Sometimes there are surprises – a kiwi, for example, contains twice as much vitamin C as an orange. And pineapples have both an antibiotic and anti-inflammatory effect. Mother Nature is simply amazing!

Squeeze me!

So how can you obtain the amazing health benefits from superfoods? Why not try your hand at juicing? Some people think this is a better way than vitamin pills to get your nutrition, as juice is easy to assimilate into the body and it's in the natural form the body can recognise. If you're serious about juicing, invest in a really good juicer. What health bonuses do you get by juicing? Well, fruit and vegetable juices are absolutely packed with enzymes, which are vital for digestion, brain stimulation and cellular energy. They're also packed with phytochemicals, which are linked with disease-busting properties. Juice is also a concentrated supply of nutrients, which juice you up with energy! And as if this wasn't enough, juices help to balance acid and alkaline in the body – over-acidity is the root cause of many health problems. Stress also produces a lot of acid compounds in the body and juices help to neutralise these.

Juicing is a great weapon in your detox armoury. Detoxing isn't a solution to every health challenge, but it can have a powerful effect on cleansing the body and establishing a foundation for health. These days however, I prefer to make vegetable smoothies using my powerful smoothie maker. In smoothies the pulp is not extracted so you get more (but not all) of the fibrous benefits of the whole vegetable. The resulting thick drink is almost like a cold soup and will sustain you for longer than a juice.

Consider taking superfoods in powder form – you can get a day's worth of vegetable requirements in one drink. The only downside is that they have an 'interesting' earthy flavour, but don't let that put you off. It could be my imagination, but I swear I feel a definite zing when I drink mine every morning!

Spare a thought for your heart

There is much we can do for our coronary health through diet, lifestyle and exercise. We also need to take account of our approach to work. Two major long-term studies, one in the US and one in the UK with civil servants have shown that there is an elevated risk of developing heart disease if we are excessively work involved and ambitious (long hours, can never 'let go'), react to pressure in an emotional manner (volatile, angry and frustrated) and are hard on ourselves (your own harshest critic).

If we do not learn to moderate our relationship with work, our cardiovascular systems may pay the price. Take a look at your relationship with work and see if you need to make changes.

- Take regular exercise to increase the general condition of your heart and cardiovascular system (your arteries and veins) – remember to monitor heart recovery.

- Do calming exercises to dampen down excessive reactivity of your nervous system, e.g. breathing, meditation.

- When under pressure, take a few minutes out every hour to allow your body to recuperate. Stress hormones (adrenaline and cortisol) gear you up for action, but can damage your body over time.

- Keep hydrated, by drinking water regularly (roughly 2 litres per day).

- Avoid excessive caffeine as this can overstimulate the brain and nervous system.

- Eat a healthy diet that promotes heart health; low fat, plenty of fruit and vegetables (particularly tomatoes, garlic, onions).

- Don't let an excessive level of work commitment and drive damage your heart!

21
Get your nutritional act together

You've made the brilliant decision to take your well-being into your own hands. Now what?

Put some solid systems in place to ensure that your good intentions actually get done. There's nothing more stressful than hundreds of 'I shoulds' running loose in your brain, like 'I really should buy fresh stuff instead of ready meals.'

My first tip is to write all these Shoulds down somewhere so that you can quit worrying about them. Break your Shoulds into sections, such as Diet Shoulds, Exercise Shoulds and Stress-busting Shoulds. Give each Should a priority rating from one to three and tackle the high scorers first. So, if 'I should stop having nine cups of coffee a day' is more of a priority than 'I should stop eating that extra square of chocolate a day', score it as a three and make it something you'll tackle this month. Only aim to take on three Shoulds a month – too many and you won't do them. Get the high-scoring ones under your belt before you take on the lower scorers.

Choose a day to start the healthy new you, but don't make it a Monday as it's always too depressing to start something at the beginning of the week, especially as the weekend is so far away. Take just one month at a time and say to yourself you'll stick to it for that month. In this way, you won't feel that what you're going to do will be forever. If you think that something is forever, you tend to rebel against it and are less likely to stick to it.

First, go through your cupboards and throw out everything with unrecognisable ingredients on the back of the pack. The general rule is get rid of any ingredient that comprises more than three syllables as this usually means that it's a chemical ingredient that might not be a healthy option. You don't have to actually throw food away, just give it to less healthy friends who don't care that the ingredients are in a kind of chemical Greek.

Once you've got rid of all the old packets of food that are lurking around in your cupboards, it's time to go shopping for the basics. You'll need some of the following essential cupboard starters to get you going:

- Organic porridge oats and millet

- Wholegrains such as brown rice

- Almonds, brazil nuts and cashew nuts

- Pumpkin seeds and sunflower seeds

- Oatcakes and rice cakes

- Tahini and houmous

- Extra virgin olive oil

- Tuna in olive oil

- Lentils and chickpeas

- Tinned tomatoes, sweetcorn, butterbeans and artichoke hearts

- Dried herbs, pepper, tamari (a kind of wheat-free soya sauce), olives, pesto, liquid aminos (a bit like soya sauce).

These are only suggestions, of course. You'll probably want to add other stuff and take away anything you don't like.

Also, load the fridge with plenty of fresh vegetables. Ones that keep are broccoli, cauliflower, red cabbage and cabbage. Frozen vegetables can be useful too, so get some peas and spinach in.

I once had a client who asked me why I'd put tuna in olive oil on the list. This is simply because I really hate tuna in brine, which I think tastes like dry old bits of wood. But hey, each to his own! If you like tuna in brine or are worried about the extra calories the oil will add, then brine it is (tuna is generally high in mercury anyway so whichever you choose don't overdo the tuna). Likewise, anchovies. If there's one thing I detest it's anchovies, but if you like them then by all means add them to your cupboard basics.

Perhaps your intentions are great, but you find that because you're working such long hours you never seem to have the time to go shopping to get good food in. If this is you then I suggest you start by taking a good hard look at your life–work balance. I hate this phrase, but it seems to sum things up here. Your life is seriously out of balance if on a daily basis you're unable to achieve even your basic shopping.

Perhaps you go at a new regime like a bull in a china shop and change everything in a week, but by week two everything has fallen by the wayside. First of all, never be ashamed if you fall off the nutrition/health horse. It doesn't matter how many times you fall off, just so long as you keep jumping back on again! Those that don't climb back on fail. So, if you mess up, just start again. Tomorrow is a new day! The other thing to do is build on your habits. A great website is Dr Andrew Weil's site at www.myoptimumhealthplan.com. He encourages small changes daily and has great recipes and ideas for exercise. Check it out as it's really, really good!

22
Think before you drink

Let's not get too hysterical about alcohol. No one's saying 'give it up'. But if you're in less than peak condition it's one of the obvious culprits.

Apparently there are heart health benefits to wine, due to the antioxidant potential (antioxidants are substances that 'mop up' cell-damaging molecules called free-radicals). Probably not quite as many as are claimed. For instance, women can only expect the benefits of alcohol to kick in after the menopause, and even then, more than one or two drinks a day is probably detrimental, rather than beneficial.

Having said that, there is even some evidence that it could do your energy levels good. A Spanish study of nearly 20,000 adults found that drinking moderately meant an increased sense of well-being and less sickness than teetotallers.

But once you get over that moderate one or two into three or four, the bad side kicks in. Less oxygen reaches your cells because alcohol causes dilation of the blood vessels. You could become dehydrated – alcohol is a powerful dehydrator. And your liver has to work hard to metabolise it if you drink to excess.

Then of course, there's the danger of hangover.

The pounding headache of a hangover is down to dehydration. Even a very slight thirst means you have already lost one per cent of your body's fluid and two cups of water are needed to replace it. When you reach hangover levels of dehydration your body is screaming for pints of fluid. Alternate a glass of still water with every alcoholic drink.

Milk thistle is a natural detoxifier that helps the liver to function optimally. Take the herb before and after drinking alcohol.

Handling alcohol on a daily basis

Let's face it, being a teetotaller is very hard in our society. For some of us, it's harder than others. I know one journalist who, when he's with his work colleagues, actually pretends to be a reformed alcoholic so no one forces him to drink. 'I just couldn't hack the amount that some of my colleagues drink and remain functioning. I don't know how they do it.' This isn't a bad strategy. He's happy to drink at home with his wife – just not with what he calls the 'booze monsters'. Here are some strategies that might help.

- Alcohol cuts down on oxygen and this leads to tiredness – both mental and physical. Don't slouch over your pint, and breathe deeply.

- Carry Nux vom – a homeopathic remedy that stops nausea and headaches.

- Watch out for high-sugar drinks like sherry and alcopops. The sugar means they're absorbed into the bloodstream faster and eliminated more slowly, so you get drunker faster – and stay that way longer. Brandy, oaked Chardonnays and young red wines may also be high in compounds called congeners that are hard on the body, their metabolism taking more energy.

- Eat before you go out – it will cut down the effects of alcohol and save you calories too. If you're full, you're less likely to get drunk, or to become a victim of 'the munchies' and start scoffing nibbles to keep going. Follow the advice of nutritionist Amanda Ursell, who recommends eating beans and toast as a stomach liner; it works really well – not filling you up too much, and minimising alcohol's bad effects.

- Your liver can process one unit of alcohol an hour. Stick to that and fill up with water for the rest of the time. You'll find you feel more in control, you may never have a hangover again and you'll have more energy the next day.

And if it all goes wrong?

Give your liver a makeover. This will help you recover your energy the day after, faster. It is best to consult an expert nutritionist before starting a supplement regime, particularly if you are on any medication, but here are some suggestions.

Take milk thistle daily. This is a herb that strengthens the outer membranes of liver cells. Research at the Cedars-Sinai Medical Center in LA shows that, if you take milk thistle in the days before a big drinking session, it reduces hangovers.

Take 1200 mg of N-acetyl-cysteine. This dose was reported by the *New Scientist* to completely banish hangover symptoms.

Take 75 mg of vitamin B complex, 500–1000 mg of vitamin C and 2 g of evening primrose oil before you go out, and repeat the morning after. This may help reduce the effects of hangover by replacing destroyed vitamins.

23
Food as glue

Why community matters when it comes to food

In ancient times, cooking and eating were communal activities but these days like many other things that were once important to us cooking has become a neglected activity. Have we perhaps lost something by spending less time in the kitchen?

In the 1950s a traditional housewife might find herself isolated in the kitchen slaving away at a hot stove while in the sitting room her husband sat under a standard lamp, sucking on his pipe and reading the newspaper with his slippers on. I remember my step-mum in the 1970s still bogged down with cooking meal after meal, for which she received (I suspect) very little thanks. Generally, until the massive expansion of the convenience food industry in the 1980s and the huge influx of women into the workplace, it fell to women, by and large, to get the meal on the table.

Through advances in technology we have been able to outsource the job of kitchen slave to the nice people at the convenience food producers. What began with frozen peas and fish fingers expanded to instant curries, vast aisles of frozen food from the supermarket (a miracle), and more recently the gastro-pub style meals from up-market frozen food stores, which promote the idea that they are all cooked fresh from ingredients that we recognise from our own kitchen.

Over the same time period how we eat these meals has changed from sitting round the table, to slobbing out in front of the TV.

We get back from work too late to prepare anything beyond something basic, or we shove something pre-prepared in the oven. We don't want to chat around the table as we've used up all our social energy at work. The kids eat separately or they would never get to bed at a reasonable time. But by eroding the old rituals of preparing something from fresh ingredients which we then sit down and share, we start to lose something very special. Eating is not only about sustaining the body, it is a visceral, instinctive, ancient, ceremonial bond that holds us, our families, our communities and sometimes even our country together.

Prioritising how we eat as a family is a way to get the so-called work–life balance back into sync. To achieve a sociable family meal you have to leave work on time. Sharing the load also helps – don't forget that even quite young children can help with simple tasks like preparing vegetables and this will also help instil in them a sense of the importance of taking time over creating a meal.

Cooking your own meals has the benefit of you knowing what is in your food (increasingly not the case when it comes to the lists of chemicals printed on the back of processed food packets or hidden in the ingredients list under harmless-sounding pseudonyms), while sitting down and eating properly aids digestion and might even help prevent common digestive problems such as IBS. Food is one of the biggest ways we can influence the outcome of our health, yet we delegate this out, and wonder why in later years we are so sick. We don't have to be sick. We can be well and happy and the choice lies in our own hands.

Once the meal is ready we need to put the technology down, sit round the table and share food in an old-fashioned way. We might just find as a family, we like each other. A shared meal is a wonderful time to download the day's triumphs and losses. Many fear that this everyday meal shared can also become a centre of conflict (with grumpy teenagers stomping off and slamming doors), but problems are much better discussed and faced here, than left to fester in the corner of an isolated bedroom.

Technology and isolation are combinations that rob us all of the ability to live life in the present, and create a host of difficulties in the long term, whatever the benefit in the short term.

We can extend the 'glue' of food out to our community, for example by buying more of our food from small, local retailers or direct from producers in the form of local 'vegbox' schemes. You're probably thinking now that fine ideas like that are all very well but frozen food from the supermarket is much cheaper. You may well be right but, as with many of our health choices, it is about priorities. Most of us can afford to spend more on healthy food if we cut back on something else. Healthy eating should not be a luxury, whereas perhaps the latest phone, your daily latte or that must-have high fashion pair of shoes are not so, well, must-have. The less stuff we feel we need, the more resources we can plough into the foundations of health – our food. Supporting our communities helps the local economy, buying locally cuts down food miles, reducing pollution, and (depending where you are) you get to know who it is that is growing your food, and an important ancient bond with your surroundings is re-established.

Food has always been about lots of really deep issues – our very survival in ancient times depended on how we could secure and store food. In times of celebration food brings us together – lots of religious celebration festivals are based on traditional foods that are eaten together. In many faiths the end of a period of fasting calls for a special meal. In the West Christmas is sometimes the only meal in the year cooked as a family, while the Jewish Passover feast is used to mark the liberation of the Israelites from slavery in Egypt. National celebrations also bring us together: for the Queen's ninetieth birthday many Brits had a giant tea party, and what meal is more important to Americans than Thanksgiving? Eating together binds us together. It is our social glue.

If you are feeling like you need to revive your relationship with food, family, friends and community try these tips for making food your glue:

1. Meal kits are becoming huge business. This is where you are provided with the recipe and fresh ingredients to make a meal, enabling you to cook the meal from scratch. Abel and Cole, among other suppliers of vegbox schemes, offers this service. It saves time thinking about what to cook and gathering ingredients together, leaving you more time to enjoy the meal with your family.

2. Keep strict boundaries between your work and home lives. The wonders of modern technology mean that we're constantly contactable but if you get a work email at 9.30 at night how likely is it that the issue can't wait until the morning when you're back at work? Keep your boundaries even if your boss doesn't.

3. Put your phone in a bowl in the hall when you come in the door and keep it switched off. If you need to look anything up, listen to music, or check your eBay bidding do it on another device not your phone. This is my daughter's tip. Technology is the killer of face-to-face real community and meaningful relationships.

4. Plan your meals.

5. Buy local – your community matters, as does your connection with your food's origins.

6. Sit down to eat together. If you are alone try not to multi-task – eat your meal mindfully (see chapter 25) before you watch the TV, read or whatever else you get up to in the evening!

If you are passionate about food how about joining a food movement? The Food Assembly is a collective that helps you source food from your immediate area. The food is locally sourced and then delivered to a local collection point. If you don't have a Food Assembly near you then you could start one. Check out thefoodassembly.com

---

24
Water babies

Seventy per cent of the planet is covered in water, and when we're born seventy per cent of us is water too. It's cool to be wet, so why aren't you drinking enough of the stuff?

There are life forms that can live without oxygen, but none last long without water. So why do we pay so little attention to it?

Do you know what constantly amazes me? People who go to a posh restaurant, spend a fortune on the meal and then think they're being clever by asking for a glass of tap water. Granted, some places seem to charge more for water than for wine, but is this a smart way of saving money? Most tap water tastes disgusting. I realise that this is my personal opinion, so do your own survey. The most unpalatable glass I ever had was in England's rural Oxfordshire. It was like drinking part of a swimming pool. Even London water tastes better despite, so legend has it, having passed through eight other bodies first. However, is changing to bottled water the solution?

Bottled bliss?

Bottled water isn't always the purest water. In fact, it might actually contain more bacteria than the tap version. Also, the labelling on bottled water makes it far from clear what you are actually getting. Most tap water, however, will contain a cocktail of contaminates, most commonly lead, aluminium and pesticides.

Generally, water can be called natural mineral water, spring water or table water. Mineral water is generally from a pure, underground source, where the rocks and earth have naturally filtered it. Spring water also comes from a filtered underground source, but does not have to be bottled on the spot. Table water is definitely the dodgiest dude of all as it's the least defined and could be a mix of water including tap water, so unless you really like the design of the bottle you could just be wasting your money. Watch out for artificially carbonated table and spring water as this can rob your body of vital minerals by binding to them, meaning they are flushed out rather than being absorbed. Also, look at the proportion of minerals – remember that salt (sodium) will dehydrate the body slightly.

Every now and then, there'll be a TV programme featuring blokes turning into women or male fish turning into female fish. Scare stories aside, the point is that we're being continuously exposed to xeno-oestrogens (foreign oestrogens) in our environment and these can have a feminising effect on our bodies. One source of these foreign oestrogens is through plastics – the worst thing you can do is leave your water heating up in the sun in a plastic bottle. So, blokes shouldn't simply blame their boobs on beer (although alcohol also has feminising effects, but that's another story!).

Water works

What are the best choices then? Well, one cheap solution is to get a filter jug, which removes the bug-busting chlorine element. The carbon filter also takes out some minerals, so another top tip is to change the filter at regular intervals to prevent manky old ones from leaching bacteria back into your drinking water. The jug should be kept in your fridge.

Another option would be to have a filter attached to your tap so that water is continuously filtered, or you might want to consider the more expensive, but definitely superior, reverse osmosis systems which separate the water from the other elements that are contained in it. This is what NASA developed for its astronauts (you don't want to think about why they're filtering water!).

Both tea and coffee are dehydrating. The diuretic effect of these beverages means that they rob the body of more than they supply. I know it's a challenge, but cut down on the amount of tea and coffee you drink. Like everything else, it's just a habit. At first, it will be a struggle but once your body realises how thirsty it is, you'll find that you'll be naturally reaching out for water rather than the colas. The phase where you need to pee more will also pass (excuse the pun), as your body will absorb the water rather than it going right through you. And since it goes through you surprisingly quickly, sipping water rather than glugging huge glasses of the stuff will help. By the way, you'll also begin to like water, rather than expecting what you drink to have flavour!

Save the oral rehydration therapy (a mixture of salts and sugar) for when you've got cholera – though some people swear by it as a hangover cure! Isotonic drinks are really intended to help athletes absorb water and energy quickly. Some are loaded with sugar – you've been warned!

If you find 2-litre bottles of water too intimidating, try the small 1/2-litre bottles instead. If you're not used to drinking masses of water, increase your intake slowly by just one 1/2-litre bottle a day at first.

25
Mindful eating

One of the great tragedies of the modern age is that we seem always to be chasing the tail of that elusive master *time.*

When it comes to eating, therefore, we are in such a hurry to get it down our necks so we can get on with the next thing that we hardly ever actually savour the food we are eating. We hardly register what tastes are there – as long as it fuels us, who cares? We eat everywhere –at our desks, mindlessly dropping crumbs down the keyboard, in the street while texting, at home in front of the TV, some of us probably even eat in the bath. No place is too sacred to cram in a few calories – then we can hurry, hurry, hurry and get on with life, and the business of being very important busy, busy people who have no time to be human. Of course all this has a cost to our health.

Digestion starts in the nostrils – as we smell the aroma of sizzling onion, the twist of fresh lime, the promise of sharp tangy mint, our digestive juices start flowing; our bodies prepare for the process of actually eating. Mindful eating is, at its most basic level, eating food with awareness, and being conscious of how that affects our bodies and our environment. When we eat unmindfully the first thing to give is our digestion. We might start to suffer from IBS, reflux, or constipation. So we rush to the doctor, hoping to solve our problem with a pill. After all, that's so much easier than actually tackling the root cause – right? But actually, if we paid more attention to the way we eat a lot of common digestive problems could be avoided.

That's because when we eat in a rush, not considering what we are taking in, we don't actually digest that well anyway. Our bodies react to our rushed state by producing stress hormones and preparing us to flee from a sabre-toothed tiger. To aid our supposed flight our digestion shuts down, so even if the food is good food, we are unlikely to absorb it optimally. In addition to that with the time-poor, cramming it in our faces method, we constantly over eat. We don't really have the sense of how much we are actually eating so just keep shovelling it in.

Many of us suffer constant guilt about the food we consume. If you're in that group mindful eating is an important strategy to get back a sense of what your food is doing for you and your body, and how it is nurturing (or otherwise) your life. Sandra Aamodt's Ted talk in 2013 and her subsequent book, *Why Diets Make Us Fat*, highlights mindful eating as a key strategy when it comes to losing weight and regaining health. Not judging is a founding principle of mindfulness, and it is particularly important to have that attitude when we eat. Noticing what we are eating, without judging, helps us make better choices.

The guy usually credited with bringing the concepts of mindfulness to the West is Jon Kabat-Zinn, founder of the Stress Reduction Clinic and the Center for Mindfulness in Medicine at the University of Massachusetts Medical School. One of the first practical exercises he gets students of mindfulness to conduct is to mindfully eat a little raisin. Normally, we grab whole handfuls of raisins and pop them unconsciously in our mouth ten at a time. In this mindful eating exercise, you just pick one tiny raisin. You place it on your hand. You look at it without judging it. You examine all its landscape, the nooks and crannies, the wrinkles and dips, the colours and textures. Then you smell it. Holding it to your ear, you squeeze it gently between your fingers and perhaps you perceive a gentle crackle? Finally, you place it in your mouth, rolling the little fellow on your tongue (no judgement remember); after a minute or two you very gently chew, releasing the magnificent burst of flavours in this tiny miracle (see chapter

60 for more on this). Of course you are not going to take every meal in with this level of detail or you would spend your whole time at the dining table, but it is certainly worth trying this exercise to fully appreciate your food and to notice your very speedy relationship with it in every day life.

In short then, mindful eating brings with it many benefits:

- Tasting food and appreciating it;

- Better digestion;

- Possible stabilisation of weight, as you consciously realise you don't need seconds;

- Enjoyment of food.

How to eat mindfully

- When eating a meal choose to eat at the table with a plate, knife and fork (or other suitable crockery and cutlery).

- If at work, step away from your desk – eat in a meeting room or dedicated eating area if available or leave the building completely.

- Vary your food choices – bring your own if you have poor choices around you, but try not to take sandwiches to work for lunch every day.

- Enjoy the anticipation of eating – smell the food and wait a few seconds before tucking in.

- Just eat – don't multitask (leave your phone at your desk, don't even take a book or paper to read).

- Savour each mouthful.

- Don't let your brain use the time for manic thinking.

- Sit for a while after you've finished eating – just a couple of minutes – rather than rushing back to your day right after the final mouthful.

26
Why you're not getting any younger

There are few things in life that are inevitable but ageing is one of them. In a way we are very privileged to be able to age, and doing it gracefully is of course even better.

In days gone by, and of course in other societies not so fortunate as our own, dying young was and is a fact of life. In the Middle Ages, you were lucky to live until you were 30. However, once you got past the major threat of dying from infection you could expect quite a good innings – until your early sixties. These days women are expected to keep batting until their eighties and even men keep going until their late seventies – with the gap in average ages between the sexes now decreasing. And some people are living substantially longer than the average. But what about quality of life? The big worry for many is how to live a great, active and healthy life until the final curtain comes down – many have seen a close relative descend into degenerative disease such as dementia. I know what this looks like up close and personal as my mother-in-law has 'mild cognitive impairment' which frankly doesn't seem very mild to me. She watches a lot of TV these days.

The good news is that our health is to a large extent in our own hands, so while the experts still aren't sure about the exact causes of some degenerative diseases, what seems to be apparent is that looking after yourself is one insurance policy worth taking out.

Typical symptoms of ageing are considered to be 75 per cent from accumulated cell damage due to our diet and lifestyle, and only 25 per cent from genetics. Anti-ageing diets are growing in popularity, leading to exciting research into their effects. What we eat and how we live our lives have an enormous impact on how we manifest our old age. Old age it turns out, is a whole bunch of biochemical processes from oxidative stress, to glycation, mitochondrial deterioration, and telomere shortening (the telomeres protect our DNA but shorten every time a cell multiplies, i.e. as we age, eventually disappearing entirely, leading to cell death). Let's take a look at each of these in turn.

Oxidative stress

These days nearly all 'healthy' products seem to say that they are 'rich in antioxidants' or help counteract 'free radicals'. We might be faintly aware that sounds like a good thing, but what exactly is an antioxidant and who or what are the free radicals?

Oxidative damage occurs when highly reactive substances containing oxygen (also called oxidants or free radicals) cause damage within the body – a bit like the rusting of the metal of an old car. These oxidants are a totally normal by-product of our metabolism – they're created every time we breathe – but also result from inflammation, infection and pollutants (such as cigarette smoke). Many experts dismiss the influence that diet has in reducing the burden of oxidation, because we do have our own enzymes in the body that mop up free-radical damage. But what has changed in the last seventy to eighty years is the onslaught of pollution from all sorts of environmental challenges and the deterioration in the quality of the average diet. And our food is getting less nutritious too. A study published in the *British Food Journal* looked at data from 1930 to 1980 and found mineral levels in produce had declined by as much as 22 per cent for some nutrients (such as iron). Another study found that you would need to eat eight oranges to get the same nutrient value that our grandparents did from eating just one orange.* Our natural enzymes have yet to catch up.

The keys to reducing oxidative stress are reducing exposure to pollutants as much as possible and increasing exposure to elements that neutralise oxidants (free radicals) – those famous antioxidants. Later on we'll look at some ways we can limit our exposure to oxidative stress while at the same time upping our intake of fresh, natural foods that are rich in antioxidants (in the form of vitamins and minerals).

Galloping glycation

Glycation is a process in the body in which glucose (the body's main fuel) binds to proteins or fats, forming something called advanced glycation end products or AGEs (I bet someone was chuffed when they came up with that one). These AGEs cause cell stiffness, and as a result over time the body's intricate communication system is made more difficult (stiff cells find it harder to transport nutrients between themselves). In the end this process can manifest as disease. Those interested in keeping their skin young will be interested to know that this process affects collagen and elastin, the two substances that keep skin firm and supple. So glycation leads to older looking skin in the form of wrinkles, sagginess and a general lack of radiance. This is an entirely natural process but we don't want to accelerate ageing or promote wrinkles where we can avoid them.

Mighty mitochondria

Mitochondria are organelles (literally little organs) inside our cells and are the power house of our energy production. These little dudes churn out energy in the form of ATP (adenosine

*   www.soil association.org/organic-living/why-organic/
     its-nutritionally-different

triphosphate) and are responsible for about 95 per cent of cellular energy production. While the process is natural and essential the by-product of producing energy is lots of free radicals which can then damage the DNA (genetic blueprint) of the cell. So the trick is to have antioxidants on hand to mop up this by-product. Guess where that comes from by and large? Yes, you guessed it, your diet. But most modern diets – those high in processed foods, damaged fats and sugar – not only fail to donate antioxidants to the system but actually create more oxidation.

Telomere shortening

Telomeres are structures at the end of our chromosomes, which help protect our DNA and ensure accurate cell reproduction. But each time a cell reproduces the telomeres get shorter and shorter (much shortening is due to oxidative stress) until they are too short to allow the cell to reproduce successfully. When a telomere becomes too tiddly the chromosome can no longer divide and this triggers cell death. Certain nutrients can slow down the process of telomere shortening; these include antioxidants, vitamin D, folate and vitamin B12. The new trends of intermittent fasting (the much talked about 5:2 diet) and calorie restriction have also been shown to help.

The big baddies

So what is responsible for causing all this damage, which we experience as the ageing process?

Sugar

This is certainly getting a bad rap these days and the discussion about its effects is not going away. It's the sneaky increase of the availability of sugar in all its forms that is a way bigger problem for our times than it was 100 years ago. Sneaky, because it crops up in almost all processed foods – not just sweet ones. It goes under many aliases and may be labelled as maltose, dextrose, fructose, syrups, or maltodextrin to name just a few – apparently there are sixty-one different ways to label sugar in the US. Sugar is added to savoury dishes to increase the 'bliss point' – the point where we say, 'Yum'.

Sugar increases the glycation process we mentioned earlier, and also increases oxidation. Alcohol (which is derived from sugar) has the same effect I am afraid, compounded by the other dangers of ingesting ethanol. Although many red wine apologists maintain that it's the best choice of alcoholic drink due to high levels of resveratrol (an antioxidant) which may buffer the effects of the oxidation moderation is definitely the key here. If you do fancy the odd glass of wine try to stick to organic red wines with no added sulphites (antioxidants added to stop the wine going off, that unfortunately don't have the same effect in your body).

Heated vegetable fats

Another trend, after years of debate, is the return of saturated fat (butter, animal fat, coconut oil). Although there is much controversy and confusion surrounding consumption of fats it looks like the big problems are trans-fats (found in some processed foods) and overheated vegetable oils. For many years polyunsaturated fats have been promoted as 'healthy' but there's more to it than that. Eaten in their virgin state they have benefits but once stuffed into a processed ready meal or cooked they spell disaster. That's because when the vegetable oils that contain polyunsaturated fats are heated to high temperatures they become chemically unstable and break down into some pretty dodgy by-products, including aldehyde and formaldehyde, which can interfere with cell programming. So avoid anything processed that contains vegetable oils (such as sunflower, rapeseed, and hemp). I know you probably know this, but it bears repeating that fish and chips and other highly fried food isn't a health food group, not only for the obvious calorific reasons but because they are often fried in this 'toxic' oil.

Pollution

This isn't only a question of what we breathe in or consume in the form of cigarette smoke (or from e-cigarettes) but what we take in through food. Conventional farming adds chemicals in the form of fertilisers and pesticides as part of the growing process, levels of environmental toxins are also increasing and we even create pollutants when we cook some foods. A 2014 study undertaken by the UK Soil Association* found that organic crops had up to 60% higher levels of key antioxidants compared to conventionally farmed versions. Another worry is that our oceans are full of pollutants which in turn end up in our fish – so although in theory fish should be healthy, the issue is complicated by the need to avoid increasing our toxic burden through fish consumption. Grilling meat at high temperatures produces chemicals called heterocyclic amines (HCA) which are known carcinogens. We need to eat even more fresh, antioxidant-rich foods to counteract these pollutants.

In short …

Oxidants, or free radicals, occur as natural by-products of your body's metabolism, or come from pollution, and dodgy stuff you eat or drink. These oxidants lead to bodily ageing. Antioxidants are like a defence force mopping up oxidants; while some are produced in our bodies, we also need to consume them as part of our diet in order to ensure an adequate supply.

That's the bad news. Check out the next chapter to find out how you can eat yourself young.

---

*   www.soil association.org/organic-living/why-organic/
     its-nutritionally-different

27
Eat yourself young

Having established in the previous chapter that we are all rusting machines that need antioxidants to stop rapid decline, what if anything can we do to slow down the ageing process?

In order to mitigate the negative effects of oxidative stress on the body and therefore slow down the ageing process our diet should be one that is high in antioxidants. These have been shown to slow the effects of cellular ageing. But it's not just about looking good – remember those little dudes, cell mitochondria, we talked about in the last chapter? They need looking after and nurturing, and in looking after these little fellows we can live a life with abundant energy and vitality – a radiant complexion comes as a bonus.

Anti-ageing foods

The major antioxidant nutrients are vitamins A, C and E and the minerals zinc, copper and selenium. But of course it's much more complicated than that! We don't yet fully understand the relationship that food has with our bodies when it is real and whole food. As humans we're inclined to think of the constituents of a food as causing an effect. But is it simply the nutrients in an apple that are good for us or the apple as a whole? What we do know is that there is a group of plant chemicals called phytonutrients that have significant antioxidant power. A diet high in plant-based foods is therefore one that is likely to be high in a range of different antioxidants. The more colour the food has ensures a good variety of these vital components, and the variation in the colour ensures you are getting a spectrum of different phytonutrients.

Getting more fruit and vegetables

A simple way to increase the quantity of fresh fruit and vegetables in your diet is to consume plenty of fresh (ideally home made) soups. Once you get more adventurous, or when the weather is warmer, you might even want to try raw soups, which will be even higher in antioxidants, since some of these fragile nutrients are lost in the cooking process.

Smoothies are also great, but make sure to include lots of green vegetables and go easy on the sugary fruits. Whole fruits contain fibre, which helps slow down sugar absorption but the smoothie-making process breaks down this fibre meaning that the sugar hit on your system is more rapid. If you add a spoonful of ground flax or other seeds it will make the smoothie easier on your blood sugar. When I make green smoothies I put all sorts of goodies in like barley grass powder, some essential fats (I like the Viridian Beauty Oil), a natural protein powder (such as Purition, which seems to be real food rather than chemicals), and then a mix of kale, cucumber, spinach – whatever's in season really. Lemon juice and an apple improve the flavour.

Herbs and spices

Herbs and spices have been found to be very high in antioxidants and have powerful properties and a high ORAC score (oxygen radical absorbance capacity). Turmeric has recently zoomed to the top of the spice charts since it exerts strong antioxidant and anti-inflammatory effects. The active part of turmeric is called curcumin and there is a great deal of excitement and buzz about it.

Fermented foods

Bliss begins in the bowel according to Confucius, and one might argue that gut problems are the root source of degenerative disease. Eating fermented foods promotes the good bacteria in our gut that keep our digestive systems healthy. Recently there has been a massive amount of research to suggest that these little bacterial passengers might have a bigger influence on our health than we ever thought possible and might even influence how our brains age too. Fermented foods include live yoghurt, kefir and unpasteurised miso and sauerkraut.

Cut the calories, increase your life expectancy

Another area of research and ageing has centred around cutting total calorie consumption to increase longevity. The aim is to reduce calorie intake by between 20 and 40 per cent. Most wholefoods are actually low in calories anyway – but the new trend is 5:2-type diets, otherwise known as intermittent fasting. This type of eating is said to imitate our ancestors' way of eating, where food was not so abundantly available as it is in our day, and may reduce the shortening of the telomeres we mentioned in the last chapter, hence decelerating ageing. In the 5:2 system one eats fairly normally for five days but calories are reduced to the bare minimum for the other two days. Another, easier, option is to do all your eating within an eight to ten hour window every day (so you might push breakfast later and dinner much earlier).

Live a chilled-out life!

All that said one of the worst things you can do is worry – it's a fine balance to be made between eating sensibly and obsessing about every little thing you consume. We evolved to handle serious intermittent threat, and that's where our stress hormones come from. But these days instead of being used to help us flee the occasional sabre-toothed tiger, our stress hormones are constantly switched on to handle everyday worries such as deadlines, demanding bosses and social pressures. We don't grant ourselves enough recovery time. Our caveman ancestors would have had a lot of natural downtime sitting round the fire or chipping away at some flints, but we need to consciously make an effort to relax. To counterbalance modern life and the stress that accelerates ageing try to spend time in nature, meditate and take regular not too strenuous exercise. Quality sleep is vital since the sleep hormone melatonin produced by the pineal gland is also a powerful antioxidant. Make sure your bedroom is dark enough, and all bright lights, technical equipment like mobile phones and computers are removed from the room at night.

Eating yourself young entails a combination of factors – reduce sugar and processed or heated vegetable fat; get away from pollution; increase your consumption of organic vegetables and real food, going heavy on the plant sources of food; include some lovely spices; lob in some fermented foods and, finally, make sure other parts of your life support recovery to counter modern stress.

Top tips for eating yourself young

- Swap sugary desserts for fresh fruit – high in vitamin C – blueberries (in season) have a very high ORAC score.

- Eat clean food – think organic, lightly steamed veg, which should reduce your exposure to pesticides and increase the number of antioxidants in your diet.

- Eat a rainbow of vegetables – red, orange, yellow, green and purple. Eating some raw food boosts enzyme intake and variety ensures you are getting a lot of different phytonutrients.

- Consider intermittent fasting. If you can't face that then maybe go easy on a Monday (after the weekend where you might have overdone it) or eat all your meals within an eight to ten hour window once or twice a week.

- Avoid cooking with vegetable oil – yes butter is back in vogue, as is coconut oil. Use fresh vegetable oils (such as flax or hemp) cold on salads but don't heat them.

- Rest is revolutionary so take quality recovery time. Yoga, meditation and spending time in nature are all rejuvenating.

28
How to eat for Wellness

Yes, yes. You've heard it all before. You are what you eat – well, strictly, you are what you *absorb*. But the truth is, very few of the people who complain of being tired are eating enough good-quality fuel to stay healthy, much less full of vitality.

There are usually reasons (let's be kind and not say excuses). We know what we should eat but … life is so crazy, we've been ill, we've no time …

I don't want to diss your doctor but, in one survey, around 75 per cent of those who went to their GP complaining of tiredness didn't get any help. GPs can help when your tiredness is due to a medical illness, but for most of us that's not the case. Yours might tell you that tiredness is hardly ever caused by nutritional deficiency and it's true that it is hard to get so low on the B vitamins that you hit clinical deficiency. But we're not eating well enough – that's a fact. Government stats show that the majority of the population is low on essential vitamins and minerals.

Some energy-boosting ideas will help even if you continue ignoring the basics, but if you don't eat well past the age of twenty-five it's near impossible to achieve everything expected of you.

On the other hand, follow the basic rules below and you will almost certainly start to feel better. All foods are equal in one way. They are broken down for fuel, but your body can use some of that fuel more easily than others. The sources the body finds it easiest to access are fruit, vegetables, wholegrain bread, pasta and rice, because these are easy to convert into glucose. Glucose combines with oxygen in the cells to become ATP (adenosine triphosphate), which is stored and used as needed. If this carries on normally all is well and we have enough energy; when it goes wrong, we are lacking in energy.

Three ways the energy supply can be disrupted

- Energy production is powered by vitamins – in particular the B vitamins and coenzyme Q10. B vitamins are relatively easy to get in the diet, but our ability to take up coenzyme Q10 diminishes as we get older. These nutrients are also destroyed by alcohol or smoking.

- Without oxygen, the glucose can't be used by the cells. Poor respiration, poor circulation and damaged blood cells (anaemia) all affect our energy levels.

- Some carbohydrates are too effective at creating energy. Refined carbs such as pasta, white bread and doughnuts are converted so quickly that if the body's given a huge dose of them – and let's face it, that's how it often gets these foods – it gets a bit overexcited, panics, and stores the glucose as glycogen. Glycogen is not so easily available as other forms of energy and also the process of releasing the glycogen takes energy, depleting energy stores even more.

So how do you use this information?

Follow these rules. They are simple, but don't underestimate how difficult it is to change habits, especially when it comes to food. Take it one step at a time.

Six-week plan to transform your energy levels

Each week concentrate on adding in one habit. You can do them all at once but, if you find eating regularly and well difficult, take it one week at a time.

1. Eat breakfast. Every day. No excuses.

2. Eat lunch. Every day. No excuses.

3. Start snacking. Never go longer than three hours without eating. Regular healthy snacks mean you don't overeat at mealtimes. Since eating huge amounts at mealtimes can deplete your energy, snacking takes stress out of your body. It also keeps your blood-sugar levels stable so you have a constant flow of energy throughout the day.

4. Add in energy-giving carbs. Eat a fist-sized portion of wholegrain carbohydrate at every meal because it supplies B vitamins and doesn't get broken down too fast; for instance, wholegrain pasta, brown rice, oats or wholemeal bread (around two slices).

5. Add in energy-giving protein. Eat a deck of cards sized portion of protein at lunch – and if you really want to see a difference in your energy levels, have some at breakfast too. That means meat, fish, eggs (2), cottage cheese, cheese, tofu, pulses.

6. Drink enough fluid – about one to two litres a day – not including alcohol or strongly caffeinated drinks.

29
Rise and dine – your energy investment

This is the one non-negotiable part of your diet! If you thought skipping or skimping on breakfast would be a good way to shed weight, you need to wake up to the fact that the opposite is true. Feast on this.

Wouldn't it be great if there was a really simple trick that made us feel full of energy and sharp as a very sharp thing for hours on end? Well there is, and it is called breakfast.

Many people give breakfast a miss because they think it will help them lose weight. New fasting regimes sometimes advocate skipping breakfast but my experience is, for working folk, breakfast is not the one to miss (if you must skip a meal consider instead missing the occasional dinner). Research has shown that breakfast eaters tend to be slimmer than breakfast skippers. This is due in part to the fact that eating a healthy breakfast keeps you feeling full for longer. That means you'll be more able to resist a quick calorie-laden snack when you're feeling faint at 11 a.m.

Studies on schoolchildren have shown that kids who breakfast show greater concentration in class, as well as increased problem-solving and verbal fluency abilities. This must also have some application to adults, as has been proven in tests on memory stimulation and breakfast eating. I expect you can guess that adult breakfasters showed superior skills in memory tests than those who went without!

What should you have for breakfast? Fry-ups are out but you can still have your bacon if you grill rather than fry it. Could you try poaching or scrambling your eggs? The best fuel combination is a carbohydrate and protein breakfast. Carbohydrate releases energy quickly (it gives you the boost to run for the bus), but protein releases energy for longer (it will help you clinch the deal during that tricky pre-lunch conference call). If you only eat carbs in the morning or nothing at all, your body may well crave more carbs at 11a.m. – hence the dreaded doughnut run that wreaks such havoc with your figure and your idea of yourself as a person in control of their life. So remember. Carbs (whole, unprocessed) good, bit of protein essential.

Cereal, whether it is based on wheat, corn, rice, bran or oats, can be a good high-fibre choice but read the label carefully as not all breakfast cereals are as healthy as they seem at first glance. Do check the label on the packet, as many cereals contain high levels of sugar. Muesli, despite its sandal-wearing, yoghurt-knitting associations, isn't always as healthy as you might think. Many brands contain vast amounts of sugar, not to mention tasty little additions such as chocolate chips. Go for sugar-free (i.e. unsweetened, not artificially sweetened) varieties or make your own. All you need to do is soak some oats overnight in some skimmed milk or fruit juice and then add some grated apple, berries or sultanas and a spoonful of yoghurt or fromage frais. You could also add a handful of nuts or sprinkling of seeds, such as sunflower. Roast these on a hot plate or a wok without oil and they will taste delicious.

Cooked oats have been around for centuries – the Roman historian Pliny recorded how early Germanic tribes ate porridge. As the starchy oats are digested slowly, porridge gives a steady release of energy that lasts for hours; it is one of the most satisfying breakfasts you could choose. The soluble fibre in oats also helps to lower cholesterol levels. Try making it the traditional Scottish way with water, it's still surprisingly good. Unprocessed, wholemeal toast with a scraping of butter or nut butter and a little protein is a good choice, too, though make sure you choose a nut butter without added salt or sugar from your health-food shop. Muffins, croissants and pains au chocolat are not good for blood sugar (see page 73).

If you can't face breakfast in the morning you are not alone, but it is important to try to get into the habit of breakfasting. My suggestion would be that you have something small and healthful as soon as you feel able. A green smoothie (better than it sounds), chunked up with a few oats would do, as would a few oatcakes with houmous. Alternatively, just snacking on fruit throughout the morning, with a few nuts for protein, won't do you any harm, as long as lunch and dinner are well balanced. Try this regime for a while, and see if you find it a little easier to eat a proper breakfast.

Although it's not ideal you could eat something on your way to work. This way you can still stay in bed until that moment when any longer and you'll be late for work. An apple and some nuts or a real yoghurt are easy to have on the go. Of course, you could always have breakfast at work. Many places of work have a small kitchen area where toast can be made, and food and drinks kept refrigerated. Be honest, will spending ten minutes to have breakfast before you start work make that much difference? In fact, it will mean you are more productive during the rest of the morning so you'll probably end up saving that time and more.

If you think you have no time for breakfast, how about getting up a little earlier, say ten minutes? OK, I can see you are getting ready to throw the frying pan at me. So how about this? Lay out the breakfast crockery and cereal, such as oats or home-made muesli or granola (see box on page 129), before you go to bed. This skims a few minutes off the breakfast preparation time in the morning. Time that can be spent actually eating breakfast. It serves as a reminder each morning to have something for breakfast too. If you have children and they are sitting down to eat breakfast, are you really not able to sit and eat breakfast with them?

How to make a great breakfast

Your staple ingredients

- Eggs – ideally free-range and organic.

- Jumbo oats.

- Milk – use oat or goat's milk if you're not having cow's milk.

- Yoghurt – unsweetened bio yoghurt made from cow's, goat's or sheep's milk.

- Rye, soda or spelt bread.

- Raw, unsalted nuts (almonds, hazelnuts, pecans, brazils, walnuts, cashews) and seeds (sunflower, pumpkin, flaxseeds, hemp, sesame). Keep these in an airtight container in the fridge to protect their essential oils.

- Nut and seed butters such as mixed nut butter, almond butter or pumpkin seed butter – available from health-food shops. Avoid peanut butter and make sure you pick a product that's free from added salt and sugar.

- Fruit such as berries or apples. Frozen fruit can also be used – berries freeze well and can be bought from major supermarkets.

- Avocado.

- Fish such as good smoked salmon and sardines (fresh is ideal but canned is more realistic; go for the ones in olive oil or tomato). Great for your energy levels.

Easy eggs

Boiled or poached eggs

Boil or poach 1or 2 eggs and have with soda bread (if not

avoiding wheat), rye or spelt toast, or Ryvita. Spread your toast with a little butter (if not avoiding dairy), nut butter, houmous, pesto (very good with eggs).

Scrambled eggs

Beat 2 eggs with a little crème fraîche, yoghurt or milk (if not avoiding dairy). Heat a little extra virgin olive oil or organic unsalted butter – don't allow this to smoke. Cook the eggs to the consistency you prefer and serve with soda bread (if not avoiding wheat), rye or spelt toast, or Ryvita. Can be garnished with fresh herbs such as dill, chives or parsley.

Scrambled eggs and smoked salmon

Make the scrambled eggs as above and add some pieces of smoked salmon when the eggs are nearly cooked. Serve on rye toast with chopped dill and black pepper. For extra protein spread the bread with a little soft goat's cheese and top with the eggs.

For those mornings when you fancy something extra with your eggs, grill or steam some tomatoes, or steam any other vegetable. Use a bamboo steamer – it takes a few minutes and is a great way to add additional colour and flavour to your plate. Try broccoli, asparagus, spinach, chard, mange tout, etc.

On toast

For a quick and easy breakfast toast a couple of slices of soda, rye or spelt bread and top with the following:

- Nut or seed butter and slices of tomato or cucumber
- Soft or hard goat's cheese and sliced tomato
- Soft goat's cheese and mashed avocado
- Tinned sardines, pilchards or mackerel and sliced tomato

- Soft goat's cheese and smoked salmon

Oats

Home-made muesli

Make a large quantity of the mixture below and store in an airtight container for a quick, delicious and economical muesli. Use one or more ingredients from each of the groups below:

- Jumbo porridge oats – use this as your base and add other flakes if desired such as rye, buckwheat, barley, millet, rice, quinoa or amaranth flakes. If you are following a gluten free diet only use buckwheat, millet, rice, quinoa or amaranth

- Mixed nuts – flaked almonds, chopped hazelnuts, pecans, brazils, walnuts, flaked coconut, etc.

- Mixed seeds – sunflower, pumpkin, flaxseeds, hemp, sesame

- Dried fruit (go easy on this because of the sugar content and pick unsulphured versions) – raisins, currants, sultanas, apricots, etc.

Combine and store in an airtight container. To serve, place in a bowl and add milk or yoghurt. Top with fresh fruit, such as berries, if desired. Can be soaked overnight for easier digestion.

Quick and easy porridge

Serves 1

2 x tablespoons of jumbo porridge oats

50 ml of water

1 x tablespoon of nuts or seed mix

Pinch of cinnamon, nutmeg, vanilla essence or ginger

Mix the oats and water in a pan and boil, reduce the heat and simmer for 1 minute. Alternatively, soak the oats the night before, in just enough water to cover them and heat in the morning. Add a spoonful of yoghurt or milk, a spoonful of the seed mix and a pinch of spice.

Very berry porridge

Serves 2

100 g jumbo oats

300 ml water

300 ml milk (or milk alternative such as soya or oat milk)

2–3 handfuls of berries, e.g. blueberries, blackberries (use other chopped fruit when berries are not in season, or use frozen berries)

1 tbsp chopped nuts, such as almonds or pecans

Place the oats, water and milk into a pan. Bring to the boil then gently simmer, stirring until the porridge starts to thicken. Pour into bowls and sprinkle the berries and chopped nuts on the top.

Apple porridge with cinnamon and nutmeg

Serves 2

100 g jumbo oats

300 ml water

300 ml milk (or milk alternative such as oat milk)

1 apple grated

1 tsp of honey

1 tsp cinnamon

1 tsp nutmeg

1 tbsp flaked almonds

Place the oats, water and milk into a pan along with the grated apple. Bring to the boil then gently simmer, stirring until the porridge starts to thicken. Add the cinnamon, nutmeg and honey. Pour into bowls and sprinkle with the flaked almonds.

Granola

Makes enough for 12 servings

500 g jumbo oats

75 g pumpkin seeds

75 g sunflower seeds

4 tbsp sesame seeds

4 tbsp poppy seeds

50 g desiccated coconut

150 g honey

100 ml extra virgin rapeseed oil or sunflower oil

Preheat oven to 170 degrees/gas mark 3. Put the honey and oil into a small pan and bring to a simmer until the honey has become runny. Place the oats in a bowl and pour over the honey and oil mixture and toss it all together. Line two baking dishes with baking parchment and divide the mixture between these. Bake for 20–30 minutes, stirring often, until the oats are golden. When the oat mixture has cooled, add the seeds and coconut and mix thoroughly. Place into bowls and serve with milk (or milk alternative such as soya or oat milk), and top with seasonal fruit.

Yoghurt

Seeded yog-pot

Serves 1

3 tbsp yoghurt

3 tbsp seeds, these can be ground or used whole (remember to chew well). Try substituting 1 spoonful of seeds for nuts.

Pinch of cinnamon, nutmeg, vanilla essence or ginger

Combine all the ingredients in a bowl and enjoy. You can also add some fruit to this such as a grated apple, chopped pear, or a handful of fresh or frozen berries.

Something for the weekend

Kipper kedgeree

Serves 2–3

225 g undyed kippers

225 g long grain brown rice

4 hard boiled eggs, chopped

25 g butter, diced

1 tsp mild curry powder

1 tbsp chopped parsley

Ground pepper

Lemon wedges

To cook the fish, place in a shallow pan and just cover with water. Bring carefully to the boil, then cover with a lid and turn off the heat. Leave for 10 minutes or until the fish is cooked through. Rinse the rice and place in a pan with enough water to cover. Bring to a simmer and cook for 35 minutes or until cooked. Drain once cooked. Skin and flake the cooked fish, checking for bones. Stir the eggs, curry powder, pepper and parsley into the warm rice. Add the diced butter and let it melt. Season to taste. Serve with the lemon wedges.

Buckwheat pancakes with smoked salmon and poached eggs
Serves 2

For the batter:

100 g buckwheat flour

150 ml milk (or milk alternative such as soya or oat milk)

150 ml water

1 egg

Olive oil

Pinch of salt

For the filling:

2 free-range eggs

70 g smoked salmon

Juice of 1/2 lemon

To make the pancakes, put the flour and salt into a mixing bowl and add the egg. Mix the milk and water in a jug. Beat the egg into the flour, adding the milk and water a little at a time to make a batter. Leave for at least one hour to rest. Lightly oil a frying pan and heat it well. Put a tablespoon of batter into the pan and roll it round to the edges. Cook until the pancake is golden then turn to cook the other side. Place the pancakes on a plate. Poach the eggs. Place the smoked salmon on one half of the pancakes, squeeze over the lemon juice, and place the poached egg on top. Fold the pancakes in half over the filling, and serve.

Buckwheat pancakes filled with berries, fromage frais and chopped nuts

Serves 2

For the batter:

100 g buckwheat flour

150 ml milk (or milk alternative such as soya or oat milk)

150 ml water

1 egg

Olive oil

Pinch of salt

For the filling:

4 tbsp of mixed berries, e.g. blueberries, blackberries, strawberries, raspberries (use frozen berries or other fruits when berries not in season)

4 tbsp unsweetened fromage frais

2 tbsp of chopped nuts, e.g. hazelnuts, walnuts, pecan nuts

A little honey

To make the pancakes, put the flour and salt into a mixing bowl and add the egg. Mix the milk and water in a jug. Beat the egg into the flour, adding the milk and water a little at a time to make a batter. Leave for at least one hour to rest. Lightly oil a frying pan and heat it well. Put a tablespoon of batter into the pan and roll it round to the edges. Cook until the pancake is golden then turn to cook the other side. Place the pancakes on a plate and fill with the fromage frais, berries and chopped nuts. Drizzle with a little honey.

Mushroom and tomato frittata

Serves 2

1 tbsp olive oil

75 g brown mushrooms, sliced

4 eggs

2 tbsp live, natural yoghurt

ground pepper

1–2 tbsp fresh parsley, chopped

2 medium tomatoes, chopped

Heat the oil in an omelette pan, add the mushrooms and soften over a gentle heat. Break the eggs into a bowl, beat them lightly and add the yoghurt, black pepper and chopped parsley. Mix well, and then stir in the chopped tomatoes. Pour the mixture over the mushrooms in the pan, spreading the filling evenly over the base. Cook over a gentle heat until the bottom of the omelette is firm. To cook the top, slide the pan under a hot grill for a couple of minutes.

30
Micronutrients matter

These days it is tempting not to give much thought to what we eat – using our busyness and budgets as an excuse to just grab the nearest and best value bit of grub. In the back of our minds most of us know that food is more important than this – but in the short term we feel OK and we don't have the time to go to great lengths cooking and preparing food. We rarely give our diets the consideration they deserve until something goes wrong. So what might we be missing out on?

It isn't just the macronutrients – carbohydrate, protein and fat – that are important, nor is it simply about the most shouted about vitamins and minerals such as vitamin C and calcium. Some of the really important players are micronutrients which are actually only needed in very small quantities – but small deficiencies can make big differences to our health. We need to consume these minerals in our food since the body can't make them.

These nutrient tiddlers do a very important job of keeping our body's machinery running. The body does a huge range of complex jobs – it produces skin, muscle and bone, it churns out red blood cells that carry nutrients all around the body, muscles are fired, chemical messages transported, instructions issued that charge your very life force. Micronutrients are the raw materials that make all these constant miracles happen. There are around thirty (discovered) vitamins, minerals and dietary components that your body needs to take in from the outside through diet.

Among this group there are a few hard hitters worth knowing more about (but of course that doesn't mean you should ignore the rest). The best advice is not to concentrate on getting more of these particular elements above the others but generally to improve the overall quality of your diet and maybe to focus on how important food is for determining your ultimate health destiny.

Zinc

Zinc is famous for being important in immunity. But what you might not know is that micronutrients can work with each other or against each other. Copper is also important in immune function but if you take hefty supplements of zinc, you may well end up depleting the levels of copper in your body and get sick anyway. This should not happen if you use zinc-rich foods rather than supplements as your mineral source. In addition to its role in immunity, zinc plays a lead role in many functions in the body, including sexual function and keeping our minds healthy.

In addition to making sure you eat sufficient zinc-rich foods you need to be aware of certain factors that reduce zinc levels in our bodies. Zinc can be depleted by phytic acid, found in grains, which inhibits zinc absorption, so you need to eat your zinc-rich foods separately from your grains. Stress is a zinc sucker, as is being ill.

Signs of low zinc can be frequent infections, slow wound healing, reduced appetite, male infertility, menstrual irregularities, dandruff and hair loss. White spots on the finger nails can also indicate that your zinc levels are low.

Good sources of zinc include oysters (hence their being famed for their aphrodisiac qualities), but these aren't to everyone's taste or budget. Fortunately other good sources include pumpkin, sunflower and sesame seeds (great for sprinkling over salads), brazil nuts, almonds, quinoa and green peas (and who doesn't like peas?).

Magnesium

While magnesium is often thought of as calcium's poor relation (if we think of it at all), any nutritionist worth their salt will tell you that magnesium is of at least equal importance since without magnesium we can't absorb calcium. Magnesium is really important to help heart muscles function and keep the nervous system in tip-top condition. It helps in the mechanism of the transcription of DNA, the body's coding, and is said to be nature's tranquilliser.

As well as adding sources of magnesium to your diet you need to avoid inhibitors. Taking calcium supplements can have an adverse effect on your magnesium levels since the two compete for absorption. As with zinc, our old foe phytic acid binds to magnesium, making it difficult for the body to absorb. And if you're partial to a glass (or three) of wine you might be interested to know that alcohol puts a downer on your magnesium status too.

If you are low in magnesium you might experience muscle tremors, spasms and weakness, insomnia, nervousness, high blood pressure or irregular heartbeat, constipation or depression, among many symptoms.

Your magnesium power-houses are kelp, almonds, cashews, blackstrap molasses, brazil nuts, rye, tofu, quinoa, brown rice, dried apricots, avocados and (in small amounts) good quality dark chocolate.

Selenium

Selenium is one of the shining stars of the whole micronutrient gang. You really don't need that much – in fact too much can be toxic – but it is an antioxidant (so it helps reduce oxidation, or 'body rusting'), protects against degenerative diseases of ageing and autoimmune diseases, slows down ageing, is involved with liver health, energy, growth, fertility and thyroid health. What a superstar!

Too much strenuous exercise, cigarette smoke, exposure to chemicals and chronic illness can all inhibit absorption so as well as including selenium-rich foods in your diet you need to avoid these inhibitors. If you have digestive problems these will also impair your ability to absorb this mineral – something even more important with a mineral consumed in small quantities than with the macronutrients.

Selenium is one of our most potent cancer-fighting allies. Reduced levels of selenium in the body can lead to oxidative damage and make you prone to heart disease. People low in selenium may experience a weakened immune system (frequent infections), hair loss, fatigue, muscle weakness, and lacklustre fertility, to name but a few symptoms.

Good dietary sources of selenium include herring, tuna (though best avoided due to its contamination with mercury), liver, soya beans (non-GM ideally), wheatgerm, wholegrains, bran, scallops, oysters, light molasses, eggs, milk, onions, tomatoes, broccoli, carrots, turnips, brewer's yeast, nuts and seeds.

Iodine

Now this next one is my personal favourite and I, along with most nutritionists, am convinced it has a huge role to play in our health. Iodine is required for good breast and thyroid health, and helps with conditions such as fibrocystic breast disease and hypothyroidism. Low iodine has in fact been associated with a higher rate of breast cancer. Japan has the highest dietary intake in the world at 13 mg per day and has the lowest rates of both goitre (a thyroid-related condition) and breast cancer. But Japanese people who migrate to America and adopt an American diet, eating just 150 mcg (that is 0.15 mg) experience breast cancer levels similar to those of other Americans. This suggests that dietary iodine plays a crucial role.

In the old days iodine was quite abundant – before the First World War we used to feed dairy cows fish meal so many people got their iodine by drinking milk (not that cows eating fish sounds natural). However, these days it is hard to eat sufficient iodine without supplementing the diet. Sea vegetables are the best source of iodine but are definitely not to everybody's taste. I supplement with a seagreens supplement (basically seaweed but in a capsule, so you avoid the seaweedy taste).

While it's relatively easy to get sufficient of these micronutrients to avoid deficiency diseases, we might not be getting enough for optimum health and to avoid chronic or degenerative disease. That's because:

- We get our nutrients through the soil (which the plants take up) and our changed farming methods over the last century have left the soil devoid of many key nutrients.

- Chemical fertilisers focus on the few elements that will produce reliable and abundant crops (such as nitrogen and phosphorus) while most plants need up to eighty different minerals from the soil.

- Pesticide use reduces the uptake of essential minerals by the plant.

- Harvesting the plant or crop before it is fully ripe is common but this deprives the plant of the essential nutrients it would get from the soil if allowed to mature fully.

- GM (Genetically Modified) plants have been shown to have reduced nutrient levels. For example, a GM tomato was designed with thicker skin, which was great for making sure that its skin wouldn't get caught up in the harvesting machinery, but unfortunately produced a fruit with less vitamin C and less lycopene than a normal tomato.

- Transportation – when foods travel long distances, or sit in warehouses, their nutrient potential diminishes. An orange can take four months from picking to land in your supermarket trolley.

- Food processing – general industrialised processes will rob the food of nutrients.

- Refining – taking a whole food and processing it for use, e.g. milling flour or dehusking brown rice, strips the nutrients out of it. This is often done to produce the versions of a product favoured by consumers, such as white flour for bread and cakes, but unfortunately much of the nutrient value resides in the discarded husk and germ of the grain in question.

We need more micronutrients than ever – the micronutrients are our defence against all sorts of elements including pollution. We need more of these little guys because we have more toxic elements in the environment, and we live ever more hectic lifestyles, filled with chronic stress.

The simplest way to ensure you have optimum levels of these micronutrients in your body are:

- Eat better quality food – invest in organic if you can afford to. Buy local. You might find it a bore but it will pay dividends.

- Avoid the nutrient robbers – sugar, alcohol, excessive teas and coffees, and foods high in phytates (processed soya for example).

- Try to choose seasonal food. That way it's less likely to have been flown miles and have lost its nutritional value.

If you are known to be deficient, you could consider supplementation but if you do, go for a quality brand, and make sure you take a balanced multivitamin and mineral supplement rather than going for spot minerals. Even better, invest in a few sessions with a professional health advisor who can tell you what nutrients you should take, in a personalised way, rather than just guessing.

31
Back to work

If you have back or any musculoskeletal problems, there are a large number of physical solutions you might want to try – a good physiotherapist, chiropractor, osteopath, or even a yoga practitioner can show you the way here. But there are also nutrients that can help you out.

Taking steps to change the cause of the issue can be obvious – perhaps you have an ancient mattress, poor desk arrangement or bad posture. In such cases changing your bed or investing in a standing desk can have a huge impact. I once knew a man who had terrible lower back problems – he visited a chiropractor who told him to remove his wallet from his back pocket (not what you think) and try sitting down. He now removes his wallet whenever he sits at his desk or in the car and his back no longer troubles him. Sometimes big problems can be caused by something quite small that you need to change or adjust. Sometimes, it's lifting something and trapping a nerve. Regardless of the cause there is no need to suffer in silence, and put up with years and years of chronic pain. In fact much can be done nutritionally to aid your recovery.

Particularly if the problem is muscular in origin, healing becomes much easier if your underlying nutrition foundation is a good one. Even your state of hydration matters since it will affect the function of your fasciae – flexible connective tissues that support muscle function and are present throughout the body. If you have tight, 'crispy', dehydrated fasciae, it makes it difficult for your underlying muscle to work very well.

So how would you rate your musculoskeletal health?

- Are you less flexible than you used to be?

- Does backache keep you awake at night?

- Are injuries ruining your exercise routine?

- Do you have signs of arthritis?

- Do you suffer from morning stiffness and/or stiffness after rest?

- Do you spend hours sitting at a desk each day?

- Do you do regular load bearing exercise?

A yes to any of the first six means you need to act now to avoid further problems. Having musculoskeletal problems is the third biggest cause of sick leave (after stress and acute medical problems – such as heart attack). Figures show that an estimated 1.2 million people suffer work-related musculoskeletal issues, and it's not just manual workers. So what causes these chronic aches and pains?

- **An extra load.** Carrying extra weight will impact how you carry your body, and how your muscles respond. It's a huge global problem – in the UK 55 per cent of the population is over-weight. People who are overweight are at an increased risk of arthritis or osteoporosis due to the increased load across the weight-bearing joints, increasing stress on cartilage and ligaments.

- **Inactivity.** Working hunched over a desk, or not living life with enough movement will contribute to our muscles not being optimal to hold up and support our frame. Use it or lose it.

- **Poor nutrient intake.** Our diet is of course essential for overall well-being. Not only will a balanced diet help with healthy weight but increasing the levels of certain nutrients helps reduce the likelihood of developing issues in the first place.

- **Inflaming inflammation.** Again our diet is a major player here – new thinking on conditions such as osteoarthritis puts inflammation down as a major contributor to how we manifest disease. Can we change that? I think we can certainly give ourselves the best possible chance of avoiding these conditions by eating in a way that promotes good health and decreases inflammatory reaction in the body. A major contributor to inflammation is an imbalance in our intake of fats, since modern diets tend to contain too many of the pro-inflammatory fats (processed foods being a major culprit here) and not enough of those that reduce inflammation, like fish oil (omega-3).

- **SAD eating habits.** The SAD (Standard American Diet) has spread its deadly tentacles pretty much everywhere. In many countries it is part of the aspirational promise of the rich Western lifestyle but the downside is that it's a diet high in glucose/fructose sugars (which is a cause of inflammation, among other things) and full of the pro-inflammatory fats mentioned above. Nauru, just off New Guinea has the dubious honour of having the fattest people on the planet, with 94 per cent of people overweight because they have wholeheartedly adopted the SAD. Adopting the SAD increases obesity, and therefore strain on the body, and encourages inflammation, both of which will heighten musculoskeletal problems.

- **Inadequate hydration.** Dehydration can affect all parts of the body especially the spine, intervertebral joints and their disk structure. The body needs hydration to lubricate joints, enabling them to sustain the force produced by weight or tension produced by the action of muscles on the joint.

- **Smoking.** Smoking increases the risk of low bone mass, low bone strength and low body weight, all of which directly impact the development of osteoporosis. Rheumatoid arthritis is more likely if you a smoker or exposed to tobacco. While fewer of us are smoking these days we need to watch the vaping too – the research isn't conclusive yet, but you are still inhaling chemicals. My bet is that vaping will eventually be found to have side-effects too. Your ultimate goal should be to kick the nicotine habit completely.

- **Alcohol.** Drinking excessively is possibly the most common health hazard on the planet. Drinking heavily has a negative impact on bone mass and contributes to weight gain, which in turn places pressure on joints.

- **Cola drinking.** Heavy cola 'use' (a revealing term used by the companies who make cola – we're more used to hearing about 'drug users') makes the body draw out calcium from the bones in an attempt to buffer the phosphoric acid that gives colas their tangy flavour. So even if you opt for a sugar-free cola (a whole other can of worms), regular consumption will have an adverse effect on your musculoskeletal health.

- **Sitting ducks.** They say that sitting is the new smoking, with a number of recent studies advising that we should move more and sit less. But for most of us there is a fat chance of that at work as we're usually deskbound. Using computers for large parts of our days is also a problem for repetitive strain type injuries.

- **Poor night time habits.** Poor sleeping posture can also be the root cause of back issues – especially sleeping on your front.

So are we all doomed to having dodgy backs, iffy knees and a future life of limping around like wounded soldiers? Well, perhaps not, if we can follow some simple nutritional advice.

Eating right for back health

The very foundation of your body's health comes from your diet. Remember, you are not necessarily what you eat, but rather what you absorb – so if you have IBS, or other digestive problems your priority should be to sort that out first or no matter how well you follow the advice below you might not be getting the optimum amounts of key minerals. Also, remember changes are best done in an evolutionary way, you are much more likely to stick to your new diet.

Always try to get your nutrients by eating fresh, great quality food. Sometimes this can seem expensive and time consuming. I get that totally. But sometimes it is about our priorities. The TV package, the flash phone, the perfect home, the latest fashions all cost money. Could it be better spent on improving your diet? Remember – health is wealth.

In general you should aim to avoid inflammatory foods and drinks such as alcohol, red meat, sugar and processed foods and eat more anti-inflammatory foods. 'Eating a rainbow' of coloured vegetables, with some fruit too, will help as will the twice-weekly addition to your diet of oily fish (though make sure it is not a polluted source – sardines are top-notch with high levels of inflammation reducing omega-3 oils and relatively low levels of pollution, and so cheap too). Fermented foods such as kefir and sauerkraut, which are becoming more readily available, are good for gut health so will help with absorption issues.

Alkalise your diet

Most Western diets are too acid forming. For optimal function our bodies actually need to be very slightly alkaline. Acid-forming foods include many staples of modern diets, such as most grains, meat, cheese, sugar, coffee and tea, and processed foods. Rather than becoming obsessive about what you eat a simpler solution is to cut back on these types of foods and start replacing them with plenty of fresh green vegetables as well as nuts, beans and ancient grains such as millet, quinoa and amaranth.

Eat the right amount of protein

A portion of protein should be similar in size to a deck of cards. Aim to eat this amount of protein at every meal. Adequate protein levels help the body repair itself and balance blood-sugar levels which will in turn help with hormonal levels in the body (but too much protein can be bad for your health). Hormones help keep calcium in the bone.

Nutrients for musculoskeletal health

The better the quality of your food the more likely you are to be getting the vitamins and key minerals you need to keep your bones and muscles healthy. All nutrients are important but we have the tendency to try and separate these things out, so here are a few key ones to help with bone and muscle health.

- **Magnesium**: Although we think about calcium for bone health, the real issue might be that we don't have enough magnesium, which is needed to help us absorb calcium. We need about 375 mg (Recommended Daily Allowance) but only get, on average, 228 mg. Signs of magnesium deficiency are muscle cramps, including menstrual cramps, problems relaxing, stiff muscles, fatigue and anxiety. Without the proper amounts of magnesium to regulate its use calcium gets 'dumped' in the soft tissues, causing all sorts of other problems. Magnesium also supports the body systems that deal with stress – and too much stress draws calcium out of the bones to buffer body biochemistry. In short, we should be aiming to up our intake of Magnificent Magnesium – and the best places to get it are leafy green vegetables, nuts, seeds, berries, seafood and dark chocolate (but go easy on this).

- **Vitamin D**: We've recently started hearing more about the importance of sufficient vitamin D in our diets, since it helps with normal development and maintenance of bone. While our bodies can make vitamin D from exposure to sunlight many of us, who work indoors all day, do not get enough sunlight, and there are of course dangers associated with prolonged sun exposure. So it's a good idea to top up your levels with vitamin-D rich foods such as oily fish, liver and eggs (the D is in the yolk). It's best to consume vitamin D with Vitamin K2 (also made by our bodies but unreliably) for which that old favourite leafy vegetables are a good source.

- **Boron**: This mineral is key in building bone and muscle and improving muscle coordination. It's found in apples, almonds, dates, hazelnuts, legumes, pears, prunes and raisins.

- **Vitamin C**: This will help strengthen connective tissue such as collagen, which is a key player in keeping everything together.

- **Supplements**: If money is not an issue and you are trying to solve a particular problem, supplements may be able to help. It is best to get all you need from the diet, and moderate your lifestyle – tablets aren't going to magically make up for poor diet and lifestyle decisions. But in real clinical need they can make an appreciable difference. For example, bromelain (extracted from pineapple) can reduce swelling, and glucosamine (amino sugar) contributes to the nutrients that keep the fluid in the joints healthy. If your diet is terrible you will probably be wasting your money on supplements since your absorption is likely to be poor, so I would advise working on the diet first and foremost.

Hydration

I have to confess I am terrible at remembering to drink enough – I really have to consciously try and remember to refuel with the water. Try a filter jug, such as Biocera, which uses a filter to make slightly alkaline water. If you, like me, are always rushing around and often forget to drink why not try setting an hourly reminder on your phone to drink some water? I keep a jug of water by my desk and in the summer add fruit, mint, cucumber and ice – delicious. In winter warming herbal teas can help you up your fluid intake.

Stress less

Stress changes your biochemistry, and can lead to calcium being leached from the bones – bones may seem solid and fixed but are actually dynamic, which means that minerals are being pulled in and out of the bones the whole time. Sleep is vital of course (melatonin, a sleep hormone, helps control inflammation). Don't forget to breathe properly. It sounds daft but focusing on breathing can really help. In biochemical terms breathing in creates more acidity in the body and breathing out creates more alkalinity, as it gets rid of carbonic acid through the carbon dioxide we breathe out. Take a look at Part 4 for some mental well-being ideas.

Exercise exercise

Get the balance right between stretching (for muscles), weight bearing for bones, and cardio. But remember some cardio exercise, such as running, puts a lot of pressure through the joints. In musculoskeletal terms a brisk walk is far better for you than pounding the pavements in your running shoes.

In short ...

- Eat right: that means real – i.e. unprocessed – food, fresh and good quality with plenty of greens.

- Sleep right: reduce stress for a wonderful night's shut-eye.

- Drink right: that means plenty of water.

- Exercise right: stretching, walking, focusing on your breathing. Remember two hours of frantic activity in the gym can't compensate for every day bad habits.

- Sit right: make sure your chair is good and adjusted properly for you, or consider a standing desk. Take plenty of breaks, walk round

Healthy dinner ideas

There is a seemingly limitless choice of ready meals, processed foods and microwave dinners available, but these are usually high in sugar and/or fat, as well as salt and chemical additives that are not beneficial to your health. Ready meals are frequently lacking in much needed nutrients, and for these reasons, a healthy home-cooked meal is always the best choice for your dinner.

Cooking a meal from scratch need not take a long time – there are many dishes that are not only relatively quick and easy to make but also delicious and healthy. If you really are pushed for time try making large batches of food at the weekend and freezing them into individual portions for quick and easy mid-week dinners. Here are some ideas to inspire you:

Quick meals

- Stir-fry with lots of different coloured vegetables. Add some strips of chicken, turkey, prawns or tofu for protein. Flavour with fresh ginger and garlic, and soy sauce, or just add oil and lemon juice. Sprinkle on sesame seeds or cashew nuts before serving with brown rice, which releases energy slower than white rice and also contains more protein.

- Piece of grilled chicken or fish. Add herbs, spices and seasonings to taste and a big plate of steamed vegetables or a fresh salad.

- Grilled lean meat or fish on a bed of couscous or quinoa, with steamed or roasted vegetables. Drizzle over a dressing of fresh lemon juice, extra virgin olive oil and cracked black pepper.

- Thai green curry made using an organic green curry sauce (healthy aisle in the supermarket) baby corn, mange tout and carrot strips. Serve with rice noodles or brown rice.

- Mixed vegetable omelette (e.g. courgettes, peppers, red onion) with a large salad.

- Chicken, prawn, or fermented, Japanese-style tofu and vegetable skewers (use red onions, courgettes, mushrooms, etc). Brush lightly with olive oil and cook under a grill. Serve with couscous or quinoa.

- Small baked potato or sweet potato with tuna, chicken or beans and a large salad. Although baked potatoes are burned quickly by the body the addition of protein means that the meal as a whole will be digested and absorbed slowly.

- Puy lentil salad (you can buy canned lentils), with chopped spring onions, chopped tomato, chopped basil and feta cheese. Serve with a large green salad.

- Grilled trout or halloumi and cherry tomato skewers with steamed vegetables or a large salad.

- Salmon fillet or chicken roasted in the oven with lots of mixed vegetables. Serve with a green salad and new potatoes.

- Cold meat (e.g. chicken, lamb or beef) left over from the weekend's roast served with a small baked potato or rice salad and a large mixed-leaf salad.

When you have more time …

These meals require more time but remember that main dishes can be prepared in advance and frozen.

- Red peppers stuffed with brown rice and mixed vegetables

(e.g. onion, leeks, courgettes, etc.) and herbs (e.g. thyme and oregano). Sautee the onion and other vegetables until soft. Stir in the uncooked rice before covering with the correct amount of boiled water according to the cooking instructions on the pack. Cut the top off the peppers and put to one side, scoop out the seeds. Once the rice is nearly cooked stir in the fresh herbs before filling the peppers almost to the top and replacing the cut pepper top. Bake in the oven until the pepper is tender. Add a slice of goat's cheese just before serving. Serve with a large salad sprinkled with pine nuts.

- Shepherd's pie with a sweet potato topping served with steamed vegetables.

- Vegetable and bean/lentil casserole served with brown rice or a baked potato.

- Vegetarian or beef chilli with brown rice.

- Chicken or beef and vegetable casserole with brown rice or a baked potato.

- Fish pie served with steamed vegetables.

- Spaghetti Bolognese with brown rice or pasta. Serve with a green salad.

- Vegetable and lentil or chicken curry. Find a good recipe and take the time to make your own curry paste rather than resorting to a jar. Add a tin of tomatoes and some coconut milk or natural yoghurt. Serve with brown rice.

- Chicken, chickpea and vegetable tagine with couscous.

There is a vast array of cookbooks out there – you probably already own a few. Why not have a look through them and highlight a few recipes you'd like to try. If you're still short of inspiration try *The Optimum Nutrition Cookbook* by Patrick

Holford, *True Food* by Andrew Weil, *The Diet for Food Lovers* by Jenny Irving and *The Kitchen Shrink, Healthy Recipes for a Healthy Mind* by Natalie Savona.

Buy a meal planner and plan your meals.

There are also loads of recipes available on the Internet; why not take a look now and cook something new tonight?

32
Sleepy snacks

It's nearly time to hit the hay and you're not tired yet. Why not have a bedtime bite to kickstart those snooze hormones? Many foods contain natural sedatives that stimulate the brain to produce calming chemicals which make you feel drowsy. Eat the wrong thing, though, and you could find yourself more awake than you were before.

A bedtime snack can not only help you drop off, it can stop you waking up in the middle of the night with a rumbling tummy. If you fall asleep easily but awaken several hours later, it may be due to low blood sugar – and a light bite before bed could nip that in the bud. You need to eat a high carbohydrate snack which has some fat just before you go to sleep. Half a banana works well as it digests relatively slowly and helps your body release sleep hormones later in the night.

To help you go to sleep in the first place, you need something that's high in complex carbohydrates, with a small amount of protein which contains just enough tryptophan to relax the brain. A bit of calcium on top of this works a treat – it helps the brain use the tryptophan to make sleep hormone melatonin. In fact the age-old sleep aid, a bowl of porridge, is probably the best sleep-inducing food of all as it contains, complex carbohydrates, calcium and tryptophan. Some 40 minutes later, your levels of melatonin will rise – setting you up for a deep, restorative sleep.

Avoid all-carbohydrate snacks, especially those high in junk sugars like biscuits – they're less likely to help you sleep. You'll miss out on the sleep-inducing effects of tryptophan, and you may set off the roller-coaster effect of plummeting blood sugar followed by the release of stress hormones that will keep you awake.

And yes, that old wives' tale about cheese before bed giving you nightmares is true. Cheese – particularly mature ones – contains the amino acid tyramine, which triggers the release of adrenaline. This stimulates your brain and can trigger vivid dreams as well as nightmares. The fat in cheese can also give you bad dreams – fatty food is more difficult to digest particularly when you're asleep as your digestive system automatically slows down. So while an army of enzymes try to break down the fat, your sleep is being disrupted and you're dreaming of being chased by a giant piece of brie.

Recipes for sleep

Try one of these healthy snacks about 40 minutes before you settle down under your duvet. This gives them enough time to perform their magic ...

- Honey with oatcakes.

- Wholemeal toast with cottage cheese (which doesn't contain the sleep disrupting amino acid in hard cheese) and pineapple.

- Yoghurt and strawberries (yoghurt contains natural sleep inducing substances called casomorphins).

- 3 sticks of celery and fromage frais (celery contains a substance called 3-n-butyl phthalide, which acts as a gentle sedative).

- Banana slices and fromage frais.

- Bagel with cream cheese and chopped dates.

- Crackers and houmous.

- Wholegrain cereal with milk.

- A small handful of nuts (almonds, walnuts, cashews) or seeds (pumpkin, sunflower, sesame).

- A few slices of lettuce – not the world's most exciting snack, but the stem in particular is full of natural sedatives

Bedtime drinks

Instead of hot milk, make this oaty alternative. Soak a level tablespoon of oatmeal in milk for an hour or so in a small saucepan. Add a large glass of milk and bring to the boil gently, stirring all the time until it has slightly thickened. Pour it back into the glass, then add a spoonful of honey and plenty of grated nutmeg. You'll soon feel your eyelids get heavier and heavier.

Very little beats a mug of warm milk and honey. But you can also try a milkshake made with skimmed milk, strawberries and frozen yoghurt or a milkshake using soya milk (soya contains tryptophan). Alternatively, make your own herbal infusion from limeflower, lemon balm and lavender adding half a teaspoon of each to a mug of hot water. Cover (to prevent the plant oils evaporating), infuse for five minutes then sweeten with honey to taste.

A simple cup of camomile tea before bed will help you sleep.

At the risk of sounding like your mum, under no circumstances drink alcohol before bed. It blocks tryptophan so all the good effects of those sleepy snacks will go to waste.

If stress is affecting your sleep try passiflora or valerian, herbs which have have been used for millennia to sedate naturally and defuse stress. They are particularly useful to help you sleep. You can buy tablet formulations that contain these herbs at pharmacies.

33
Restful sleep

Do you sleep like a log or are you about as relaxed as a rather angry ant colony?

Personally, and rather annoyingly I sleep like a log – I've trained myself over the years not to think too deeply about anything close to bedtime. Some of our sleep problems come from our mental approach to sleep – an inability to let go of stress and worries for example, some come from outside forces such as our environment, and some come from our underlying health and nutrition. Of course, sleep will seriously affect your work performance and even your ability to conduct your job safely. You probably know if you're not sleeping as well as you could be but have a look at the little questionnaire below and see how many you answer yes to:

- Do you often have problems getting to sleep?

- Do you often wake up during the night?

- If so, do you wake up with a racing heart?

- Do you frequently wake up feeling the need for more sleep?

- Do you snore?

- Do you often suffer from fatigue throughout the day?

- Do you always rely on coffee/tea or caffeinated soft drinks to keep you going throughout the day?

If you answered yes to any of these questions you probably

need to make some adjustments to your diet and lifestyle before you fall victim to serious illness. To begin with it might help to understand why sleep is so important.

Unbelievably scientists aren't 100 per cent sure exactly the role sleep plays. It does seem however that a lot of repair and processing takes place at night. Recently, the experts seem to have discovered that during the night the brain's 'cleaning staff' get to work, hoovering up damaging debris called protein plaques. One study at Johns Hopkins Bloomberg School of Public Health in Baltimore found that getting less sleep or sleeping poorly was tied to an increase in brain levels of beta-amyloid, the toxic protein that builds up and forms plaques in the brains of those with Alzheimer's. They can't currently work out if poor sleep causes this protein build up or whether poor sleep is the symptom of this protein build up.

Dreaming may be the brain's way of processing the day's events, like defragging a computer hard disk – the current thinking being that the brain cannot possibly store all the enormous amounts of information taken in during the day. We'd go potty if every tiny experience was floating round our heads. How would we store information for recall? It would be like trying to find one tiny piece of information if you were one of those people who hoarded every newspaper they'd ever bought. According to sleep expert Professor Jim Horne, the brain rests and recovers in about five hours so, allowing for sleep cycles, seven hours sleep should be enough, but there do seem to be individual variations. We all know that when we don't get enough sleep we are not completely rational.

If you are having sleep problems there are some simple, practical steps you can take to make your lifestyle and bedroom more conducive to a good night's sleep.

- Make sure your room is really dark, and cool.

- Switch off the wi-fi at the router (some people really are sensitive to it).

- Remove your phone and other electronic devices from your room and try to avoid using a screen of any kind for at least an hour before bed (the bright lights disrupt your body's wind-down process, meaning you'll take longer to get to sleep). Some phones have a night setting which takes the blue light off – but phones aren't a good idea as they are too stimulating.

- Make sure your room is neither too hot nor too cold. In general to get a good night's sleep our body needs to experience a drop in temperature, but modern, well-insulated houses are often too warm. So turn that radiator thermostat down in the winter and keep your window ajar in summer if you can.

- If you wake up in the middle of the night avoid looking at the clock. Lying there calculating how many hours you have until you have to get up is not going to help your relaxation. So put your alarm clock somewhere out of sight.

- Go to bed and get up at the same time every day to give your body a chance to get into a regular sleeping pattern.

- Don't stress if you do miss out on a few hours of sleep. The idea of a continuous eight-hour stretch of sleep is relatively modern. In the Middle Ages they got up and said a few prayers after a few hours sleep and then went back to bed. If you're lucky enough to work for yourself you might find this pattern works for you. Just don't use those inter-sleep hours to do anything that's going to leave you wired.

Once you've sorted out the logistics of sleep there are of course lots of nutritional ways of ensuring you get more good quality shut-eye.

Avoid blood-sugar lows

Our human engine runs ideally on average on about 1.5 teaspoons of sugar (glucose). You might not think that we need very much fuel at night but the brain is a big consumer of glucose and any repair mechanisms operate on glucose too. It is surmised that when blood sugar levels crash during the night the body reacts by releasing various stress hormones such as adrenalin and cortisol to drive the levels back up by breaking down supplies stored in the muscle and the liver. The only slight snag is that this sudden surge wakes us up with a pounding heart, and sweating palms. These crashes are more common when alcohol or processed foods, which turn into sugar quickly in the body, are consumed in the evening. Balance your blood sugar by eating nutrient-dense food that releases its energy slowly (see Chapter 15).

Choose sleepy dinners

Choose dinners that will help you sleep, not ones that leave you tossing and turning. Eat a small portion of good quality protein with plenty of fibre (which helps slow down the speed at which sugar is released into the bloodstream) and good quality slow release carbohydrates – so vegetables rather than pasta or rice. Eating earlier in the evening so you don't go to bed feeling full also helps. I try to eat with my daughter between 6.30 and 7 p.m. these days, which gives me plenty of time to digest. It's usually best to avoid spicy food late at night.

Kick the caffeine

It may sound obvious but it bears repeating: don't go for caffeinated drinks. If you must drink coffee have your very last one of the day directly after lunch – remember that the residues of caffeine in the body can last for as much as 14 hours in some people. Naturally caffeine-free alternatives include redbush (rooibos) tea and fruit or herbal teas. It's hard to find adequate alternatives for coffee but there are some pretty good instant drinks on the market made from things like barley and chicory. They might be worth a try if you have a big caffeine habit and can't stomach another camomile infusion.

Avoid tyramine-rich foods

Hard cheese really can disturb your sleep, and give you strange dreams or even nightmares. That's because it is a source of tyramine, an amino acid (one of the building blocks of protein) also found in higher levels in smoked meats, ham, sausage, aubergines, potatoes, tomatoes, peppers, sauerkraut and chocolate. Tyramine is thought to increase levels of noradrenaline, a stress hormone which in larger quantities inhibits sleep.

Enjoy tryptophan-rich foods

Tryptophan is converted to serotonin which makes the so-called sleepy hormone melatonin. Scoffing food high in tryptophan ensures you have enough raw material to make melatonin. Increasing tryptophan can help with low mood too since it is used to create the 'happy hormone' serotonin. The snag is that you need to eat the tryptophan food with enough of the right type of carbohydrate, which helps the tryptophan to be delivered in the cells. Some people say that there should be a time lag too between eating the tryptophan rich food and the carbs but in any case eating a protein food with a slow-burn food will balance the blood sugar so you will be achieving something even if the ideal amounts of tryptophan aren't being delivered. Tryptophan-rich foods include: bananas, figs, dried dates, cottage cheese, eggs, milk, halibut (yes, a bit random), beef, turkey, seaweed.

Good sleepy bedtime tryptophan snacks include:

- Oatcake with cottage cheese (which unlike hard cheese does not contain tyramine);

- Rye bread with a slice of good organic turkey;

- Egg and oatcake;

- Eat foods with calming nutrients.

Calcium and magnesium work together to help relax nerves and muscles. We are often chronically magnesium deficient however – signs of magnesium deficiency can be indicated by insomnia, muscle cramps and weakness (including menstrual cramps) inability to relax, fatigue and anxiety. Leafy green vegetables are full of magnesium, but be aware that because of modern farming the levels have really dropped in the last 50 years. You might consider supplementing about 400mg of magnesium. (Calcium intake is not normally a problem but we don't always absorb it efficiently; magnesium aids calcium absorption.) Sources of food containing both magnesium and calcium include: nuts and seeds, green veg, fruit, berries, and seafood. For more on magnesium see page 137.

34
Food and mood

You rarely realise how stressed you are till the day you chew the head off a shop assistant for taking too long at the till. However, when you do lose your cool like this, it's time to admit you've got a problem. Clever food choices can help.

Up until the point you really lost it, you probably thought it was the shop assistant with the problem. After all, they're the one who can't count the change without moving their lips, right?

Be careful how you voice this problem. Well-meaning friends and family members will suddenly get ultraconcerned. They tell you to relax, take it easy, breathe deeply, go out for long walks. You smile through gritted teeth. Don't these people know how busy you are? You have no time for all this namby-pamby relaxation nonsense. You have to get on.

Stress is dealt with in various chapters in this book, but right here, right now, is there anything you can do to elevate your mood? At least so you don't snap at friends when they give you all that advice on de-stressing.

What can I do?

Well, one thing you can do immediately is balance your blood sugar levels. Don't panic! Put thoughts of diabetes and daily injections out of your mind. You can do this through what you eat and once you've got the hang of it, it's like falling off a log.

We all have to balance our blood sugar levels to a greater or lesser degree, depending on how our body handles the sugar (glucose) in the blood. Very simplistically, sweet things or fast energy-releasing foods will send your blood sugar levels soaring high like a rocket and then crashing rapidly down again once the hormone insulin rushes in to lower the sugar in the blood. The trick is to choose foods that sustain you. Dense, fibrous foods such as lentils do this rather than sweet or starchy foods like gluey white loaves of bread, or potatoes. Eat slow energy-releasing carbohydrates, with or without protein, which will raise blood sugar levels slowly.

So, what effect does wildly fluctuating blood sugar levels have on mood? Well, in case your partner hasn't told you already, this can make you irritable, grouchy and fatigued. Not great things to aspire to if you want to handle your stress better.

Allergy, allergy everywhere

Food intolerances, referred to by some as food allergies, seem to be all the rage these days. Generally speaking, an example of a food allergy is if you fall down gasping when you eat nuts. A food intolerance can have loads of different effects on the health, but you may feel anything from a general unwell feeling to aching joints. It may also affect your mood. If you suspect you might have a problem then visit a nutritionist.

Fat head

Omega-3 and omega-6 fats are called essential fats because they are. Essential that is. Your body's hormones and your brain run on them – the brain is more than 60 per cent fat – so make sure you're getting enough. It is thought that although today we get sufficient omega-6 fats, getting adequate omega-3s is trickier. This creates the wrong balance between the two fats. Sources of omega-3 fats include flax seeds and oily fish like sardines, mackerel or salmon.

Food and mood

An easy way to improve how you deal with stress is to reduce the amount of tea and coffee you drink. These contain stimulants that only make you more hyped-up and tense. Try cutting down on those lattes and see how you feel.

If you thought that tryptophan was a village in Wales, I'm afraid you're wrong. Tryptophan is an amino acid (protein building block) that can help raise levels of the mood-boosting neurotransmitter serotonin. Foods high in tryptophan include figs, milk, tuna, chicken, seaweed, sunflower seeds and yoghurt, but you need to make sure you have plenty of B vitamins in place for your body to process it (especially B3, B6, folic acid and biotin). You also need vitamin C and zinc. Eating some slow energy-releasing carbohydrates with a tryptophan-rich food also helps your body process the tryptophan and turn it into serotonin.

Eat several snacks during the day rather than three great big meals. This will prevent too many massive peaks and dips in your blood sugar level so you'll be able to step off that blood sugar rollercoaster. Choosing the right kind of food to snack on is key. Although snacking itself is controversial I've found working people tend to need something to keep them going or they are just too hungry at the end of the day, causing problems like diving into the biscuit tin, crisps or vino when they get home. So on balance a healthy snack is the better option. Protein is low on the GI index and doesn't just mean great slabs of meat. Snack on nuts and seeds – almonds and sunflower or pumpkin seeds are ideal. Or try oatcakes with goat's cheese, houmous or cottage cheese. And if this doesn't appeal, fruit with yoghurt is always an option.

35
Stress-free supplements

Managing stress is simply a matter of managing your body's chemistry. There is a whole battery of supplements that can help you do this.

They can give much-needed support to help your body fight off the worst ravages of stress when the going gets tough.

If your diet is absolutely brilliant then you might not need a vitamin and mineral supplement – but I doubt it. Food just ain't what it used to be and some people believe that our soil is not producing food with the same high nutrient content that our grandparents enjoyed. Even if you eat the sort of exemplary diet full of whole foods and never touch processed garbage, we face more stressful lives than our forebears – and stress 'eats' up the body's nutrients. Those who have recently been ill, those who have undergone surgery, those who smoke, drink alcohol or regularly run for a bus (suffer any regular stress, in other words), will all probably benefit from taking a good-quality multivitamin because all of these situations stress the body, and when the body's stressed it rips through vitamins and minerals.

But there are special occasions when extra help could be useful.

If you have had a shock, or know that you are about to go through a stressful period – getting married, sitting exams – think about investing in a B-complex supplement. This supports the nervous system. Your body can't store B vitamins and has to replace them every day (which is also the reason you won't overdose on them, though of course it's sensible to follow the instructions on the bottle).

Stress affects your immune system and if you seem to be getting every bug going, you will probably benefit from an antioxidant supplement. Vitamin D is the big one – it acts almost like a hormone and helps regulate the stress response. If you're worried you can buy simple finger-prick tests to check your levels. You can then supplement according to your requirements. Vitamin C is a powerful antioxidant that has been shown to help the body recover from shock faster. (When patients were given antioxidant vitamins following trauma or surgery the mortality rate was 44 per cent lower among them one month later than in a group of patients not given antioxidants.) Consider taking a vitamin C supplement two or three times a day. Around 500–1000 mg in total should be enough; don't go over 2 g a day and don't take large doses of vitamin C if you have a history of kidney stones.

Herbal healers

Your pharmacist or local health-food shop can give you information on herbal supplements that help when you're stressed. Always talk to your pharmacist or health professional before buying herbal supplements. Some interfere with prescription drugs. When it comes to herbal help, the best supplement to reach for is ginseng. It is one of the herbs that Russian scientists first dubbed the adaptogens – 'substances designed to put the organism into a state of non-specific, heightened response in order to better resist stresses and adapt to extraordinary challenges'. In other words, it helps boost performance, which is why athletes take it in the build-up to a big competition as it helps prime the body to operate at its peak in stressful (especially competitive) situations.

How ginseng works is still unknown. It's thought it might affect the part of the brain called the hypothalamus, which controls the adrenal glands. By supporting the adrenals, it reduces the amount of stress hormones produced. Thus, ginseng minimises the effects of stress on your body. Herbalists recommend you take ginseng for no longer than three weeks without a break as it loses its effectiveness over time, but there are formulations that are designed to be taken all year round that clinical research has shown do some good in defusing stress and boosting energy. Ask your pharmacist for guidance.

Finally, there's another herb called rhodiola that is very good for helping you gain focus and concentration under stressful conditions. Students who took the herb for 20 days outperformed those taking a placebo, were less tired and felt less stressed. Like ginseng, if at all possible, start taking it a couple of weeks before a stressful period.

Zinc is very good for combating the effects of stress. Look for a supplement that combines zinc with the main antioxidant vitamins A, C and E. This is a good one to reach for when you're really up against it.

Make sure you choose a high-quality supplement in order to benefit. Many of the supplements sold on the high street do not have sufficiently high levels of the active herb or mineral to have an effect. Spend a little more and try a high-quality brand (see the Resources section on page 333).

36
Eating to beat the blues

Sometimes we all feel only a family-size chocolate bar or packet of crisps can make us feel better. But comfort eating doesn't have to mean binges and elasticised waistbands. Learn how to exploit the relationship between your diet and depression.

Bodies need many nutrients to generate the brain chemicals that influence our feelings. Want a diet to max your mood? Include these essential nutrients but go easy on unhealthy foods.

Sweet nothings

You don't need a book like this to tell you that when you eat something sweet, you get a head rush. But have you noticed, about an hour after that fifth doughnut, feeling as if you're going to pop, then sleepy and perhaps even a teensy bit irritable? Why? When our moods dip, many of us reach for sugary foods or some so-called 'refined carbohydrates' like white bread, white rice and processed foods. You're not going to like it but time-honoured comfort foods give you mood swings. Another problem with these products is that they perpetuate craving cycles. When blood sugar levels fluctuate wildly, this overstimulates glands, mucking up your hormones and worsening depression. No prizes for realising being fat and spotty won't do much for your self-esteem either. Craving balance? Eating small, evenly spaced meals keeps your blood sugar levels and your mood steady.

Taking a tryp

Tryptophan, a building block of many proteins, has been used to treat depression successfully. Not so surprising if you know your brain has many naturally occurring chemical communicators. One of them is serotonin. When we're depressed, we have lower serotonin levels. Tryptophan is converted into serotonin in our bodies. Foods rich in tryptophan include: turkey, chicken, fish, pheasant, partridge, cottage cheese, bananas, eggs, nuts, wheatgerm, avocados, milk, beans, peas, pulses, soya milk, pumpkin seeds, tofu and almonds. Unfortunately, as tryptophan is just one building block and because it's fairly big, others that are more easily absorbed by your body will be taken up instead. The way round this is to divert the competition by eating starchy foods, like brown rice, wholemeal bread, porridge oats and jacket potatoes in the same meal as tryptophan-rich food.

Omega-3

Depression is about ten times more common in Europe and North American than in Taiwan. In fact, depression is pretty rare in places like Hong Kong and Japan where they eat a lot of fish. Scientists thought this might be because depression is related to omega-3 fatty acids, which are found in fish oils. Researchers investigating omega-3 supplements have found it helps severely depressed, even suicidal patients. Fish and seafood provide the complex omega-3 most important to the brain. Don't eat fish? I'm afraid you'll need to count on your body converting a simpler fat called alpha-linolenic acid (ALA), into omega-3. The easiest way to include ALA in your diet is by munching nuts and seeds. Walnuts, brazil nuts and flaxseed are your best bet. And go organic. Organic milk contains 70 per cent more omega-3 than standard milk.

Iron man

If you're low in iron, you'll be tired and less likely to be up for any mood-boosting exercise. Rev up your iron stores by putting some red meat on the table at least twice a week. Roast beef, venison and calves liver are all good sources. Vegetarian diets can be very healthy, but the key here is balance, particularly when it comes to iron and vitamin B12. Low levels of iron will make you feel tired and sluggish, which could pull your mood down, while vitamin B12 is essential for brain function.

Microbiome

No, not a visitor attraction in Cornwall, though it does have something in common with the Eden Project. Your gut is its own microenvironment and as it turns out this little world is vital for mental health. Look after your friendly bacteria and they will take care of your mood. Eating real, unprocessed food is a good way to help maintain the correct micro-environment.

Now you know the basics you can combine some mood-enhancing foods and create a delicious gourmet treat, like wholemeal pasta with tuna, cheese and pine nuts, to make your mouth water and mood soar.

37
The inconvenient convenience food truth

As we trade in our time for money we lose something very fundamental: our absolute connection with our food. It is only since the industrial revolution that we, by and large, have been outsourcing the production of our food to others on a large scale. As people abandoned the tough rural life with its swings of fortune between famine and hardship, for the promise of a better life in the cities with the mirage of permanent work and money, workers had to buy their bread and other provisions from people they no longer knew, and possibly shouldn't trust (as you probably know, all sorts of undesirable additives were used to bulk out Victorian food to make it cheaper for the provider at the ultimate cost to the consumer).

As our working habits have changed, from the 1960s onwards, with more women working, less time spent in the kitchen, more time-saving equipment and the emphasis on food as fuel rather than social glue, we have had to place even more trust in others when it comes to what we are eating. The role of family nutritionist is one that most families have neglected to fill. For some of us our nutrition planning might stretch to a last-minute perusal of the fridge on the way out to work to identify whether someone needs to buy a few things on the way home. But many of us don't even get that far. At the end of a long working day, there aren't many hands-up for getting stuck into chopping the onions and cooking from scratch. Of course, I am generalising horribly and perhaps you cook every night, but sometimes it's really hard to do that, especially as there is often little thanks for being chief chef and bottle-washer.

So we have outsourced this little problem to one of the many supermarkets which have created products to serve our every need. We shop industrially (i.e. without any connection to where our food comes from) and resort to buying prepared food, because it's easier and seems cheaper to do so. For most food manufacturers the priority is to keep us happy so we buy their products and keep coming back for more. Unfortunately this is easily achieved by tossing in sugar, even in savoury meals where we might not expect it, which is both delicious and addictive, virtually guaranteeing a repeat purchase. It's easier than cooking our own food (this time we're trading money for time), and there is a perception that fresh food is expensive, while prepared food is relatively cheap.

Recently we have become more aware that processed food might not be terribly good for us, so to protect their revenues manufacturers have started creating product myths. Food is packaged as lovingly prepared, home-made, pastoral, natural, organic and wholesome, with the good ingredients pushed right to the fore and the less desirable ones hidden in the small print on the back of the packet (guess what – organic sugar is just as bad for you as the conventional sort). There might even be a picture of 'Farmer Giles' (part played by a model) or an artist's impression of 'Loch Ramoch' on the pack (I just made that up so if you want to use it to sell your steaks you are going to have to get my permission).

Realising that we are a bit suspicious of ingredients lists that read like a chemistry set some manufacturers have taken to the practice of 'clean labelling', where new, palatable names have replaced the chemicals. Rosemary extract might make us think of something lovely and fresh but it's actually an antioxidant preservative derived through chemical extraction.

We only have to think about the horse-meat scandal that rocked Britain a few years ago to realise how little we know about what is in these packets of food. It was found that a substantial amount of horse meat had been added in to pre-packaged food labelled as beef (and other meat). Eating horse is perfectly acceptable to many people and would be fine if you had gone out intending to buy a horse-meat pie, but you are being conned if you go to buy a beef pie and end up with one containing some old nag. Not good at all. That begs the question: What else don't we know about our food and the folks supplying it?

When food is processed it is nothing like the same as when you cook a meal at home. There is a lot of chemical window dressing that goes into making your shepherd's pie look like it was 'lovingly prepared' from 'natural' ingredients – it's a re-coloured, taste-improved, texture-tweaked and enhanced illusion. But it's far worse than simply being conned – this pretend food might actually be a major contributor to your illness pathways. It's simple: you cannot choose health and eat processed food.

Two cracking books do this topic far more justice than I can in a few pages. The first is Felicity Lawrence's book *Not on the label* and the second is the more recent *Swallow this* by Joanna Blythman. A major investment in how we buy and prepare our food is needed and waking up to how we are being conned is a major start.

Try these solutions when convenience food seems the best option. I realise these are variations on a familiar theme (it shows I'm in earnest):

1. Look at your work boundaries. Is your time for money being traded fairly or could you get some time back for health by making a clearer divide between home and work?

2. Plan your meals and organise your grocery shopping rather than eating by accident.

3. Try a recipe box so that delicious raw ingredients are

delivered to your door hand-in-hand with a recipe, all ready for you to do the cooking. If it seems expensive at first glance try your current habits for a few weeks, and keep a track of costs, and then try the boxes. You might be surprised to see you save money. It's a huge growth market – I'm not the only person to see the value of these boxes – so there are plenty to choose from, but I can vouch for the Abel and Cole boxes which I regularly buy myself.

4. Grow your own stuff. I am no gardener but for the first time I am growing a few things in a raised bed this year. The pesky slugs have eaten my courgettes! But I love the reconnection I have with just growing stuff. Honestly it is a miracle that pleases me every day. I live in a city so this is on a tiny scale ,but growing and tending your patch, however small, relaxes you and connects you to nature, and of course you know exactly what's gone into your meal. Yes of course we will eat whatever the slugs will allow us but that will keep us going for about a week – it's not The Good Life (self-sufficiency) yet. Although I am seriously considering chickens.

5. Get all the family engaged! The other day we cooked from a recipe box and all the family did a little bit of it; it was fun and we got it done in half the time.

38
Optimising immunity

Our immunity to illness is one of the most important side-effects of maintaining balance in our lives. In order to have a healthy immune system you need to get the right combination of rest, joy, laughter, sleep, nutrition (of course) and exercise (just right and not too much).

The immune system is really complicated – and made up of loads of different components and processes. The immune system works as the body's defence system and is constantly on alert to identify and destroy anything that threatens to attack the body and cause illness – viruses, bacteria and toxins. This defence system includes the physical barrier of the skin, specialised white blood cells, antibodies and friendly bacteria in the gut.

The immune system's main job is to recognise what belongs in the body and what appears to be a foreign body (antigen) like a virus, bacterium or fungus. As antigens try to breach the body's defences various soldiers are called in to fight off the threat. White blood cells constitute the intelligence and communication network that organise the response of the immune system to decide what specialist help is required. This 'army' is standing by in various parts of the body (tonsils, adenoids, thymus, spleen, lymph nodes, appendix, bits of the small intestine, and the bone marrow). There are loads of specialised blood cells all with different jobs, such as switching on or switching off immune response or blasting invaders to kingdom come. T-lymphocytes, B-cells, macrophages (hoovers of cellular debris), mast cells (which create the immune reaction), killer T-cells and helper T-cells, a dynamic duo of invader destruction – all do their job in fighting off illness.

So what are the top tips for keeping your specialised army in tip-top shape?

Look after your good bacteria

A healthy human gut will have over 1.5 kg (3.5 lb) of probiotic (good) bacteria, with more than 400 different strains, these probiotic bacteria outnumber our own cells by ten to one. Creepy thought – we are not ourselves but hosts to loads of bacteria!

These bacteria are everywhere – mostly in the colon but all over the place – you name it, from in our mouths to our armpits (as anybody who has spent time on the underground on a summer's day with someone else's armpit bacterial colony shoved in their face will know only too well). These guys keep our body in balance and protect us against the harmful bacteria. Washing with gentle soap, trying to steer clear of harsh chemicals helps ensure our bacterial colonies stay healthy. But taking care of the friendly bacteria in your gut is the major strategy. Those small dudes love fermented foods such as sauerkraut, kefir (fermented milk), kimchi, miso and pickles, which are all becoming more readily available. Fermenting your own vegetables is also pretty easy and there are plenty of recipes on the internet. Perhaps you might consider a good probiotic with the advice of your nutritionist or your local independent health food store.

Eat a rainbow of wholefoods

Well you don't need me to tell you this one. Fresh, colourful and preferably organic vegetables are rich in vitamins, minerals, fibre and antioxidants which ensure your own immune army is well fed and full of nutrients to kick some butt when those invaders attempt to breach your defences. Let them try.

Avoid immune depressors

Stress, excess coffee and tea, cigarettes, alcohol, sugar and refined and processed foods rob the body of nutrients while giving it nothing in return. Although antibiotics can save our lives, they can also wipe out our immunity by indiscriminately killing off the good guys too. Approximately 70 per cent of our immunity resides in the gut. Excess use of antibiotics can leave us prey to opportunist infection, and our misuse of them is leading to more bugs that are resistant to antibiotics. On 11 December 1945, at the end of his Nobel lecture, Alexander Fleming, who discovered penicillin, sounded a dire warning. 'There is the danger', he said, 'that the ignorant man may easily underdose himself and by exposing his microbes to non-lethal quantities of the drug make them resistant.' It hasn't taken long for this scenario to become a reality. So only take antibiotics if you absolutely need to, don't let anyone push them on you for conditions that would naturally just heal themselves and make sure you use them as instructed.

Get smelly!

Garlic and onions are naturally anti-viral and anti-bacterial. When I was travelling in China a few years back, I regularly noticed people popping whole garlic cloves before eating as a kind of preventative treatment for food poisoning. That tactic doesn't gain you many friends, but your immune system will thank you. You might consider taking a supplement of allicin, the active ingredient in garlic.

Increase immune-boosting nutrients

- Vitamin A is an infection-fighting vitamin vital for the health of the mucous membranes – like those found in your lungs. But you can have too much of a good thing – don't take the retinol type of vitamin A if you are pregnant or trying to conceive, and never exceed 10,000 iu a day.

- Vitamin C is needed for antibody production. It's relatively safe since what it doesn't need your body simply excretes – but for this reason doses of as little as 1 gram can cause stomach upsets (it's different in everyone and some people can tolerate as much as 3g). Don't take high doses if you are on the pill or pregnant.

- Vitamin E helps mediate antibody response and works with selenium to improve resistance to infection.

- Vitamin D, which triggers and arms the T-cells, is produced by the body as a response to sunlight. However, if you live in northern climes or spend much of your time indoors it's very tricky to keep enough in your body over the winter months. Your doctor should be able to test you if you think you may be deficient – you can supplement with D3 (a type of vitamin D) – I use an oral spray by Better You, which tastes lovely and is quick and easy to remember to do.

- Zinc is an antiviral mineral that promotes healing and is needed for the production of antibodies and fending off infection (see page 136).

- Selenium is another important antioxidant nutrient which protects against free radical damage and degenerative disease (see page 137).

- Turmeric contains an active ingredient called curcumin which is anti-viral, anti-bacterial and anti-inflammatory. People with seriously compromised immunity swear by this bright orange herb, which is part of the same family as ginger. Many nutritionists believe that turmeric is best absorbed in the presence of fat and black pepper. (Only today someone told me that she has a home-made turmeric tea daily. She puts two heaped teaspoons in a mug with black pepper, coconut oil –another superhero – and a little hot-water. Lovely.)

39
Stress-free eating

In this mad world we are always whirling from one activity to another – we fill our lives to the brim. The whirling and the busyness in themselves aren't destructive, but our expectation of what we can fit in to a limited time, the pressure we put upon ourselves to achieve it, makes us stressed.

I always think that in modern life we can't possibly compare ourselves to people living in London during the Blitz or medieval peasants scubbing around searching for scraps of food. How can we say we are stressed when we have food and homes and death isn't raining from the sky? But according to a recent survey modern folk are likely to be kept awake or stressed by a whole host of issues including terrorism and rising house prices. Added to that stress is the way we work, most of us, desk-bound, without seeing the sun, hunched over a keyboard, working through lunch while stuffing a sandwich in our mouths – we just don't do enough to counteract the effects of this unhealthy pressure.

For some people this tips into downright exhaustion. We keep running on empty and then our health starts to suffer. As a nutritional therapist I see a lot of patients in this condition, the symptoms of which include (but aren't limited to):

- Feeling exhausted;
- Lack of drive (including reduced libido);
- Cravings for salty foods;

- Low blood pressure (a sign of long-term, chronic stress), or high blood pressure (a sign of acute stress);

- Sleep problems;

- Digestive disturbances;

- Weight gain.

The stress hormones we produce are extremely powerful and while they were useful for caveman life, in modern life too much of this hormone being stimulated all the time can have a damaging effect on the body. Just the right amount of stress (positive pressure) keeps us motivated, but too much can drive us into the ground.

So how well do you cope with everyday pressures? Try this mini stress questionnaire:

- Do you get ill when you are on holiday?

- Do you have difficulty sleeping?

- Do you often feel unrefreshed when you wake up in the morning?

- Is your blood pressure higher than 120/80?

- Do you clench or grind your teeth?

- Do you become dizzy when you stand up suddenly?

- Do you get a second wind when you stay up past 10 p.m.

- Do you feel sleepy mid-afternoon?

- Do you perspire easily?

- Do you often feel angry about/and unable to cope with small things?

If you answered yes to 5 or more of these you might have a functional health condition called 'adrenal fatigue', not necessarily serious in itself but a warning sign that you should start to take care of yourself before your symptoms worsen and you do start to experience chronic health problems.

So what can be done?

There are quite a few nutritional and other things you can do to start improving your stress and fatigue.

Balance your blood sugar (that old chestnut)

What you eat influences how you manage your energy in the day. If you are getting dips in blood sugar your body will use other hormones to boost your levels. Eating food that stabilises blood sugar will even out how stressed you feel and may help to improve your mood. (See page 73 for more details)

Cut the caffeine

Caffeine increases production of stress hormones, and worsens blood sugar fluctuations. Caffeine can stay in the body a lot longer than you may think (as long as fourteen hours) so it might be influencing how you sleep even if your last cup was at lunchtime.

Embrace the healing power of herbs

Some herbs are helpful for short-term use when we are undergoing periods of stress:

- Ginseng. There are several types of ginseng, however four can be helpful in reducing stress, Siberian, Korean, Panax and Indian or Ashwagandha ginseng are all good at normalising the body in times of stress.

- Maitake is a mushroom that grows in clusters at the base of trees and has been used for thousands of years in Chinese medicine as a herb that helps moderate the immune system.

- Liquorice root, an adaptogenic herb (which means that if you are stressed it brings down stress hormones and if you need more oomph it can help with that too), is said to help with the hypothalamic–pituitary axis (which helps regulate hormones). Liquorice is said to boost energy, but at the same time calm the mind.

- Lemon balm is a sedative and tonic herb that calms and regulates the nervous system. It's easy to grow in a pot in your garden and can be used to make a delicious soothing herb tea.

- Passion flower has a mild sedative effect. It is said to relax blood vessel spasms, reduce the severity of migraines, promote sleep and help combat anxiety, insomnia, depression and nervousness.

Other helpful herbs are valerian, lavender, hops, Kava Kava and camomile. If you are interested in pursuing the herbal route why not pay a visit to a good herbalist, who will create a personalised herbal prescription for you.

Keep calm and breathe deeply

Breathing deeply completely changes your body's biochemistry for the better by adjusting the levels of carbon dioxide in the body. Breathing is the bridge to the parasympathetic nervous system – the bit of the nervous system that switches things off. So breathing switches off 'alarm' and promotes almost immediate calm. Breathing has been used, for thousands of years, as a focus in meditation. Focusing on breathing can stop us overthinking situations and catastrophising, and help ground us in the present. Even just a couple of deep breaths can help to change mind-set, and refresh the spirit.

Eat food contaning stress-busting nutrients

I know I keep saying it, but eating a diet bursting with freshness and stuffed full of the goodies that nurture your immune system can give you a great general foundation for health, vitality and calm living.

- Magnesium helps in the relaxation of muscles and can be found in green vegetables, broccoli, parsley, rye bread and brown rice to name just a few (see page 137 for more on magnesium).

- Calcium – helps with nerve and muscle function. That doesn't mean you can go stuffing your face with cheese though; healthier sources include green leafy vegetables, legumes, figs, oranges, sardines, almonds and tofu.

- Vitamin D – is needed for bone and immune health but the stress hormone cortisol may disrupt vitamin D uptake. If you're under a lot of stress try getting outside a few times a day to take up the odd ray of sunshine (ten minutes here and there rather than baking yourself to a crisp) to make sure you keep up your levels of this essential vitamin. That short break from your desk will also help reduce the stress.

- B vitamins are really helpful for the nervous system; they are found in lots of foods but oats and brown rice are particularly good sources.

- Chromium, which helps balance blood sugar is found in chicken, eggs, fish, potatoes and rye bread

- Vitamin C is used by the adrenal glands (where your stress hormones come from) and this vitamin is 'sucked' up quickly during stress by these little glands so make sure you get plenty of vitamin C-rich fruit and veg such as peppers, green leafy vegetables and kiwis, when you are under pressure.

- Zinc is used quickly by the body in periods of stress, but is needed for healthy muscle function and the immune system. Famously in oysters it can also be found in liver, eggs, red meat, pumpkin seeds and mushrooms (see page 136 for more on zinc).

Finally, running away is always an option when you get too stressed. Stress is part of our 'fight or flight' response. If there is a way to avoid the source of stress why not take it? Einstein said, 'A clever person solves a problem. A wise person avoids it.' Remember, he who fights and runs away, lives to fight another day.

40
Your resilience foundation

'It's a mad, mad world,' seems to be a theme of mine – but I genuinely think that in some areas we have completely lost the plot.

We want more and more stuff to fill our homes and satisfy our senses and in order to achieve that we have to work longer and longer hours. We barely even give a second thought to our bodies, and what we put them through in order to achieve this. We kind of assume that our body is separate from our head, which we assume is the real us, and we don't really pay attention to them until they 'let us down' and we find ourselves ill. And then we are a little cheesed off. We complain about our bad backs, limpy legs, diabetes or dodgy heart. What we haven't taken in, is that all these problems are by and large completely avoidable through lifestyle and diet. There is always the potential for bad luck involved for some people but much illness is unnecessary. We 'head people' have spent so long hunched over our computers, so long thinking, so long relying on technology, so long believing that we are not actual animals and are above really doing what serves the complete us, that we've failed to notice that our bodies have had enough. They are checking out.

Our bodies are a reflection of our selves, our health, our mental well-being – everything. You only have to look at a child who is sad to see how that emotion has captured their whole body. Our bodies have intricate biochemical feedback systems that influence mood. For example smiling will release endorphins, which are both natural mood boosters and painkillers – it turns out that smiling helps us stay healthy as by releasing these chemicals, the immune system is boosted. Reshaping our downturned mouth to a smile releases serotonin, a neurotransmitter that acts as a natural antidepressant, changing our outlook from negative to positive like the flick of a switch. There is a catch – it has to be a genuine smile that uses the eyes (the Duchenne smile) or it doesn't work properly.

So we can influence our health through our body and attitude – but what about our genetics, aren't we limited by the hand we are given? Controversially, the outcomes of our health might not be completely down to how our genetics have dealt the cards. It is thought that what we bathe our genes in, in effect our environmental soup, is vitally important. The emerging field of epigenetics, a scientific discipline that looks at the non-genetic influences on gene expression, gives us hope that in looking after our minds and most crucially our bodies, we can achieve resilience (the ability to bounce back) not only mentally, which is where most wellness programmes in companies focus, but physically, which we all tend to ignore.

Mental resilience feeds into physical resilience and vice versa. The key is to realise that when our head feels out of sorts the cause may be either physical or psychological. We are not designed for modern life – in many ways we are still cavemen. As comedian Ruby Wax (no stranger to mental issues) says: 'We are not equipped for this century, it's too hard, too fast and too full of fear; we just don't have the bandwidth. Our brains can't take in so much information in a world where we're bombarded by bad news and force-fed information … you open a newspaper, everyone's dead. We are only supposed to know what our neighbour is up to; if the woman next door to you is having sex with the man next door to her we need to know; but four doors down, and it's none of our business.'

'One of the greatest shortcomings of human logic is the unquestioned belief that psychological problems, be it of behaviour or intelligence are influenced only by psychological factors and that physiological problems are influenced by physiological factors. This presupposes ... that mind and body are two different things.'

– Dr Carl Pfeiffer

Only once our basic needs are met can we move on to achieving our true potential. (Psychologist Abraham Maslow's famous hierarchy of needs says all sorts of basic needs have to be met before self-actualisation or achievement can occur.) This self-actualisation could be said to equate to resilience. We can't bounce back if we don't have any food, shelter, safety, belongings or esteem or if we are under threat. But once we have these needs covered, and look after ourselves with our own resilience foundation of great quality food, sleep, focused minds, and movement – well, perhaps we can bounce back or weather whatever life has to throw at us.

Your nutrition resilience foundation plan

As a nutritionist I always start with food. Here are just a few things you can do to help increase your resilience.

Look at the quality of your food – the power is in the quality

Making sure your food is the best you can possibly afford maximises your micronutrient intake, enabling you to bounce back from illness (or even avoid it in the first place). We know that having inadequate levels of vitamin C can cause scurvy but inadequate levels of other nutrients can contribute to all sorts of conditions and disease. Zinc is very important for mental well-being as is the B group of vitamins. So quality is king. I know I've said it many times before, but look into local, organic food and where possible prepare it yourself (see Chapter 30 for more on micronutrients).

Respect your gut – it's amazing

An emerging area of study has been looking at the microbiome (the environment of your gut) and the role it plays in keeping us healthy on all sorts of levels. Seventy per cent of our immunity comes from our guts but it turns out there is an intricate feedback mechanism between our gut bacteria and our brains. Some inhabitants of the microbiome release neurotransmitters, just like our own neurons do. So don't settle for IBS, or any other type of issue with your gut. Change your diet. Do what it takes for you to take your wellness into your own hands. Eat fermented foods. Cut the sugar. Increase the fibre from natural foods. Consider a probiotic supplement. Go and see a nutritionist but don't accept that you can't do anything about it (see Chapter 14 for more on digestive health).

Balance the blood sugar (yes, that old favourite)

Dips in blood sugar can seriously affect your mood and effect all sorts of hormonal influences in the body. Eating real, dense, wholefoods will help (for more detail on this see Chapter 15).

Nurture your neurotransmitters

I mentioned serotonin earlier and these neurotransmitters (brain chemicals) are all ultimately created from what you eat. Serotonin is made from tryptophan which is an amino acid (found in protein foods). But serotonin production is not as simple as eating a load of turkey (a good source of tryptophan), we also require 'cofactors' to bring about the biochemical reactions that create serotonin. For this we need plenty of zinc, B6 and B9 (folic acid) so need to eat foods rich in these vitamins and minerals. One more thing on this though, it looks likely that the artificial sweetener aspartame is a serotonin antagonist (it works against it). Another reason to stick to real food. Dopamine is another neurotransmitter, involved in our sense of reward and pleasure. L-tyrosine (another amino acid) is converted first to L-dopa and then to dopamine and requires vitamins B9 and B6, zinc, nicacin (vitamin B3) and ferrous iron in its production. Abuse of drugs and addictive substances influences the production of dopamine, but you probably already know that cocaine isn't a health food.

GABA is yet another neurotransmitter that plays a part in calming you down. Vitamin B6 helps with its production. Acetylcholine is an important body chemical that transfers nerve signals from one nerve ending to another – it is derived from choline (found in high quantities in meat, fish, dairy and eggs) and also needs B6 for its production.

Looking after your brain means paying attention to what you eat. Food is not just fuel, where anything will do. A few years back there was a big trend for protein diets. They had the positive effect of creating well-balanced blood sugar, but by focusing on just one element of body chemistry many followers of the diet were neglecting others. Many were eating too much protein, protein of poor quality, and had terribly unvaried diets. Anecdotally, some people just ate sausages. It doesn't take a genius to see that cannot be healthy. (Now the trend is more good fat, by the way.)

So while there are foods that are particularly high in tryptophan or L-tyrosine or choline the best way to eat a diet that nurtures you is to look at it holistically, rather than wasting nutrients stressing about what precise combination of foodstuffs to eat or breaking it all apart and analysing exactly what does what.

Restorative relaxation

As human machines we need to make sure that we find the off switch from time to time. So making sure you take quality downtime is essential. Stress drains out important resources and leaves you less resilient. Making sure you have enough magnesium, found in leafy green veg is very important. Magnesium aids good sleep too (see Chapter 39 for more on eating to reduce stress).

41
Making time for health

If everything is going our way and life is floating along on its own little peaceful cloud, isn't it easy to be a virtuous health princess or prince? In that ideal scenario there is acres of time to get to our PIYO class (fanatical mixture of Yoga and Pilates) or to consult our Zen Master and grow all our own organic food in our window box, before checking in with our earth energy – and that is just the morning's well-being activities!

There are two things that scupper our best intentions on the path to vibrant health; and the first naughty little scupperer that gets in the way of all our good intentions is that four letter word that most of us who haven't yet won the lottery have to get down to eventually, if we want to eat that is. What is it? Yes, you guessed it, W.O.R.K.

Unless you work for yourself, or in a job where you can choose your hours, you are confined in a working hour routine that is not defined by you. Your work hours are generally dictated by who you work for and what industry you are in. Unless you do shift-work or are a farmer, you are generally going to be working inside, within daylight hours. In winter that can mean you are never outside during daylight, ensuring you miss out on vitamin D-making opportunities, and leading many of us to feel SAD during the dark months of the year.

Brits are meant to have the longest working hours in Europe – although consistently the French, who work shorter hours, are more productive – which suggests it might be worth paying attention to what our Gallic chums do.

With all those hours being sucked up by a greedy workplace it doesn't leave much time to actually live the life bit. The so-called work–life balance has always struck me as a bit of a misnomer. You are in your life whether you are at work or not. It's always your *life*. The long hours and lack of time to nurture yourself mean that if you haven't prioritised getting basic health fundamentals in place, when pressure strikes all your good intentions are shoved out of the window. Which leads me to the other four letter word: T.I.M.E.

Time rules our life. Time gets eaten. Time flies. And we run out of time because we let work get in the way – we haven't created the structures to support us in keeping us healthy and well. We push ourselves, we steal sleep in order to fit it all in. Many of us wouldn't plan our work the way we plan – or don't plan – our lives. We don't put sufficient priority on ourselves – instead it's just one more email, just one more meeting, just a quick catch-up on social media. Then we realise we have missed the gym window, eaten too late because we didn't get round to buying our groceries (takeaway – just this once, for the third time this week), and have been sitting on our behinds for ten hours straight (back problems again?). So how do we go about creating structure?

The first thing to realise is that the structure will not be magically created fully formed. It evolves, so be patient with yourself. I am far from perfect, but here are a few of the structures and tips which help me stay on course. Adopt the ones that work for you, adapt some, add a few of your own and keep on evolving those habits so that they give you a framework when every type of obstacle is in the way of you succeeding.

Eating structure (part 1)

The first sensational thing I discovered was a simple menu

planner – I have a magnetic one that goes on the front of my fridge. It's a bit old technology – pen and paper – but I find that works best for me. You can inspect the fridge, look at your diary commitments for the week, and by comparing the two, can write into your planner what you are going to cook each day. With a bit of clever fridge husbandry you can often make a meal stretch over two days rather than cooking a completely new meal each day. This sensationally cuts down on both waste and cost. It may not sound much, but the menu planner is the difference between successful eating and having the pizza delivery boy on speed dial. You might find it hard to get into the habit to begin with but don't worry about being perfect. I find setting aside a time to plan, normally on Sunday evening, helps. You know that is your dedicated time to plan your week.

Eating structure (part 2)

I know this sounds like an expensive option, but I am a nutritionist, so I prioritise investment in the food part of my health structures. I order from an organic company that delivers weekly. Part of my order is 'recipe boxes', which contain both the recipe and the freshly sourced ingredients to cook a delicious meal. This means there is no waste – for example, when you go to the supermarket, or indeed get a regular veg box, you probably buy several carrots, but in the recipe box you just get the one carrot you need. It might be a little more expensive but what you've spent in money you will save in time – perhaps as much as two hours by not having to go to the supermarket. It's also cheaper than reaching for the phone and ordering a takeaway. And it works really well with the menu planner. When I compare my food budget and the amount of wasted food to that of my friends, I am leagues ahead.

Exercise structures

I am lucky to be able to spend money on a trainer once a week

– but I recognise this is not the most cost-effective solution for most people. And in any case this kind of one-to-one coaching is not for everybody. Having to turn up for an appointment keeps me accountable.

There are plenty of apps, books and other programmes out there that you can use to help your exercise structure. I recently bought a PiYo CD starring Chalene Johnson. It comes with a chart that keeps you on a schedule, something I find works for me. She's quite tough!

If you plan a workout increase your commitment towards it by getting your kit ready the night before. So I have the CD, CD player, mat and workout clothes all ready before I go to work, or however upset Chalene might be that I haven't shown up to my session bed's always going to seem like the better option when I get back from my day. My trainer, Ben, is so hardcore that he's just able to stick to his fitness plan by telling himself that it is 'non-negotiable'. After a while it simply becomes habit – which is what I mean when I talk about giving your structures the chance to evolve.

Space and time structures

1. Switch off your phone. Free yourself from manically checking it.

2. Book a class (yoga, guitar lessons, Spanish conversation, whatever) at a time just after work so you know you have to leave on time.

3. Make time for mindfulness. If you find it difficult to meditate on your own try a class or download the Headspace app for mindfulness. Check out Bill Harris at Centerpointe who has a CD series, or visit Jack Black's MindStore.

Now decide what your structures are going to be. Make sure your exercise clothes are clean and ready and that your trainers are by the front door? Can your dog keep you accountable by scheduling in walk time? Are you going to start by planning your food? Or is your priority setting boundaries around work or technology? Whatever it is for you, and even if it is one tiny thing, you will find that having a non-negotiable block in your life will help keep you fit, healthy and ready for anything.

Part 3

Exercise your way to Wellness (even if you think you don't have the time)

42
Why exercise makes you feel on top of the world

You may hate the idea of it, but taking exercise is life-changing. Once you get into the exercise habit, you won't want to stop.

The reason that so many of us are put off formal exercise as adults is a hangover from childhood: unless you were good at sport at school you probably detested PE.

At school there was cross country running on a cold winter's morning, followed by a cold shower. As you get older, however, you need to give exercise another chance. There are loads of different ways of exercising and it doen't have to involve being shouted at by an angry man in a tracksuit with a whistle (unless you want it to).

The key to incorporating exercise into your life is to find something you enjoy. There's something for everyone. Some of us love swimming. For others, it's running or tennis. These days gyms have a huge variety of classes on offer, ranging from the highly choreographed to gentle classes featuring very simple moves. There's no excuse for at least not trying some of them out. If you really don't like gyms, there is walking, which is a very good exercise indeed. It is easy to get into the habit of taking regular walks. Just one foot in front of the other, walk out of your door and keep going.

Why bother to exercise? Here are five compelling reasons

1. Exercise fires up the metabolism, it builds up muscle, which burns up more energy than fat tissue.

2. Exercise gives you a buzz. You've probably heard of the runner's high, that happy, almost euphoric feeling during an exercise session. Experts put it down to a combination of factors – a release of endorphins, hormones that mask pain and produce a feeling of well-being; the secretion of neurotransmitters in the brain that control our mood and emotions and a plain old sense of achievement. Whatever gives you the high, there's no doubting the feel-good glow it gives you.

3. Exercise boosts your confidence. Every time you work out or play a sport, you're doing something positive for yourself, which is mood-enhancing in itself. When you start to see the results in the mirror, your self-esteem rockets. As soon as you see results, you will find it easier to stick to your weight loss plan, too.

4. Exercise reduces your appetite. Recent research has noted that both anaerobic exercise (such as weight-lifting) and aerobic exercise (such as cycling, swimming or running) suppress the appetite-stimulating hormone ghrelin. Aerobic exercises also increases release of the appetite reducing hormone peptide YY. The bad news is that you will need to exercise quite intensely for about an hour for this effect to kick in, although some appetite reduction was noted at lower levels of exercise.

5. Exercise really can be fun. Depending on what you choose to do, you could discover a whole new social circle. I know a few people who met their partners on the Stairmaster at their gym! Don't imagine that everyone else at the gym will be gorgeous. Only the very expensive gyms are stocked with

beautiful, thin and rich people – the heaviest weights they lift are their Louis Vuitton bags. Avoid them unless you're looking for someone beautiful, thin and rich.

43

How to start exercising when you really don't want to

Research shows that when life gets busy, exercise is one of the first things to get bumped off the schedule.

But before you berate yourself for your lack of sticking power, it's good to remember that, even for professionally fit people like personal trainers, exercise is cyclical. There will be times when it gets pushed to the sidelines. However, for those who have learned how much exercise helps them cope with a busy life, the gaps before they start exercising again are likely to be shorter than for your average Joe. If you've never exercised at all, this idea aims to get you to a stage where you too know that the benefits are so great, it isn't worth going without it for too long.

This idea is equally suitable for those who have never exercised regularly, and those who used to, but have lapsed. If it's too easy for you, ratchet up a gear, or jump some steps – but beware. Research has shown that there are two reasons that exercise programmes fail:

- we don't see the results we want (that's dealt with below); or

- we set our expectations too high.

It's far better to do a little and stick to it until you have the exercise habit, than go nuts, join a gym, write an ambitious exercise programme and then give up completely after a couple of weeks of failure to keep to it.

Decide on your goal

If you've never exercised before, or haven't for a long time, please start with a modest goal. If it's ten minutes of activity a day – that's brilliant, as long as you are confident you will do it. Aim to visit your local pool once a week, then three times a week. Aim to swim once a week, and walk round the park once a week. Aim to do a yoga class on a Saturday morning.

You gotta have a plan

You need to make a schedule where every week you are aiming to do a little more, a little more frequently until you are exercising for around three to four hours a week – enough to get you out of breath for most of the time. That could take a year, but don't think about that now. Stick your monthly schedule on the fridge. At first your goal should be just to stick to your weekly plan. Once you've got the hang of it, you can make your goal bigger, such as: run round the park, undertake your local fun run, cycle to the next town then cycle back.

If you are very exhausted, very unfit, have been ill or are very overweight, all you might be able to manage is walking up the stairs. Fine. Make that your goal: to walk up stairs three times a week, then five times a week, and so on from there. Aim for cardiovascular exercise to begin with, that gets your heart beating, because that's the type that will give you energy fastest.

If you haven't exercised for a while, try this programme.

Week 1   Walk slowly for five minutes, walk briskly for five minutes, walk slowly for five minutes. Aim to do that for three days a week.

Week 2   Aim to do the same five times a week.

Week 3   Walk slowly for ten minutes, walk briskly for ten minutes, walk slowly for ten minutes. Aim for four times a week.

Week 4   Walk slowly for five minutes, walk briskly for twenty minutes, walk slowly for five minutes. Aim for five times a week.

Then start running for blocks of time. Eventually, you'll be running for most of the time and doing it every second day.

When you're drawing up your plan, remember the acronym FIT: frequency, intensity, time per session. First work on frequency – aim to do some form of exercise five or six times a week. Then work on 'T' – the time you spend at it each time you do it. Then move on to the intensity – use hills to make you work harder, or go faster, or try a more difficult stroke if you're swimming.

You might also want to try one of the many great apps out there that help you plan and execute your exercise regime, or treat yourself to some wearable tech to help you track your progress.

Try to put the idea of losing weight out of your head. Studies have shown that those who exercise with the goal of losing weight are far more likely to give up. Why? Because you have to exercise really pretty hard to see weight loss – about six hours of running at a moderate pace every week. Concentrate instead on making it your goal to get more energy. You don't have to exercise anywhere near as hard to achieve this. You'll get results a lot sooner. If you start exercising again, specifically to feel better about yourself and get more energy, you'll find you feel excellent in a week or so, and that's more incentive to keep going. Then you can think about cutting calories.

44
Out there and doing it

I hate the gym. So, what are the alternatives?

I hate the music in gyms. I hate the smell of them. I don't like the machines and they don't like me. I only have to attempt to trot on the treadmill and I find myself getting spat off like Wile E. Coyote in another failed attempt to catch the Roadrunner!

I just don't think the gym is beautiful. And, on top of that, no one talks to each other because they're so busy doing exercise. OK, I know that's what you're supposed to be doing, but still. It's all those mirrors, too. Everyone is so busy being narcissistic and it's so dehumanising – loud music, bright lights, functional, high speed. You're in and out of there with no connection to the rest of the human race. The other obvious thing wrong with the gym is that you join up and then don't go for a whole year. When you finally do go, out of guilt, you spend a wad of cash in accumulated membership fees on one swim. Sorry, I'll stop ranting, but did I mention that I don't like the gym?

Getting it where you can

So, what other possibilities are there? Go and exercise outside. You don't have to be in the midst of the glorious countryside for this one. Your local park will do. Use the park benches to stretch, use steps to run up and use lampposts as distance markers. Let your imagination run wild as to what you can use in the environment to help you in your mission. Set goals – a good one might be to count the number of times you run round the park, each time trying to improve upon the last. I had a great little run that I used to do by the River Thames in London (down by Chelsea Harbour) where you can see loads of wildlife, cranes, fish, swans and ducks, despite being in the city. What a pleasure. Now I live near the coast and can run on the beach – even better!

Getting some aerobic exercise by running and walking will obviously increase your cardiovascular fitness, and even in the city (away from busy roads) you'll benefit from breathing 'fresh' air into your lungs. Pumping your heart muscle is important to get your lymph system moving – your lymph has no internal pump. The benefit of aerobic exercise is that it is thought to protect you against all sorts of nasty diseases, including some types of cancers and heart disease, plus it makes your bones stronger. So, get out there and do some cardiovascular stuff. Run, jog or walk for at least 20 minutes each day.

Power walking – Stride out when you walk. Get into it by loading your iPod up with some seriously good music.

Jump higher – Skipping is a wonderful way to get your ticker really going. Apparently, jumping rope has the calorie-burning capacity of jogging. But you have to really go for it – no weedy jumping allowed.

Warm up and wind down – Don't forget to stretch at the beginning and end of your workouts. Warm, stretched muscles are muscles that are less likely to be injured.

45

Get on yer bike

It's difficult to injure yourself cycling because it's such a low-impact form of exercise, plus it's a great way to tone your legs and the nicest way to see the countryside.

Cycling will also strengthen your heart, lower your blood pressure, boost your energy, burn off extra fat and reduce stress. So, what are you waiting for? Get on yer bike!

Stretch it out

Some cyclists, particularly those of you who hop on your bikes and cycle to work, rarely bother to warm up. If this is you, you might want to take a long hard look at your flexibility and posture. The main thigh muscle (the rectus femoris) has a high chance of being damaged unless you stretch it out properly. Another thing to watch out for is tight hamstrings and pulled hip flexors (at the top of the front of the thigh), which can happen if you don't take time to stretch. A heel dig stretch might help as a basic exercise to help all three of these common muscle problems. Simply lift your toes, keeping your knee straight and your heel on the ground, until you feel a pull in the back and front of the calf and upper thigh.

Hunching at the handlebars can lead to a permanent rounding of the shoulders and back. A typical yoga exercise can help counteract this – the Cobra. Lie on your front with your arms by your sides and lift your chest and head until you feel the movement in your back and shoulders. Don't forget to cool down properly too. Don't come to an abrupt halt, since your blood will pool in your legs. Instead, slow down gradually and finish with a few minutes of the heel dig stretch.

Getting the right bike for you

Your choice of bike depends on what you want your bike for. Mountain bikes are rarely suitable for riding in town and that goes for racing bikes too, however flash they may look. Having your head down when you ride is a sure way of going headlong into a bus! If you've splashed out on a new bike, consider getting it sprayed with nasty black paint in order to stop other people thinking what a beautiful new bike you have and stealing it.

Swallow saddles are back in vogue. These are long pointy saddles with an unfeasibly small sitting area that must owe more to aesthetics than to comfort as I imagine it's akin to sitting on a knife. Look for a seat that has a three-layered saddle of gel/foam/ elastic that reduces pressure on the prostate and pubic bones. Aaah, that's more like it!

Getting the right gear is paramount to making you feel safe. Wearing a helmet is vital – most accidents on bikes resulting in serious injury involve unnecessary head injuries. Also get yourself a bright fluorescent jacket or a reflective strip. Back and front lights are the law, but make sure they're good ones – it's all about being seen. Don't ride along hugging the curb, as this will encourage cars to ignore you. Within reason, own your lane so that cars have to make a conscious effort to pull out and pass you properly, like they would another car, giving you plenty of space. When you're passing parked cars, keep a particular eye out for people suddenly opening their car doors, another good reason for allowing plenty of room around you when you ride.

Get some good lightweight waterproofs so you can cycle in all weathers. Nowadays you don't have to look like an angler expecting a force 12 gale as waterproofs are made of extremely lightweight material, which folds up into a very small bundle. (Peake do good gear.) Get both top and bottoms and even consider waterproof shoe covers. Clear goggles are also a good idea, as they'll stop water or stones being flicked up into your eyes. You might not look beautiful with all this gear on, but you'll certainly be dry!

Indoor cycling

If the weather is not conducive, get an indoor turbo-trainer for your road bike, thereby enabling you to watch an engaging DVD or listen to some motivating music, while you exercise. Some of the better trainers even allow you to monitor your progress. Indoor cycling really helps your regime; it's safe, it's not weather dependent and you can stop anytime without having to walk home! Hitch yourself up to a heart rate monitor and keep your beats per minute at your optimum. Also monitor your heart rate recovery; improving this vital sign is a measure of heart health, as well as fitness (recovery of about 30 bpm from peak heart rate is the ultimate goal, e.g. peak = 146, 1 minute later = 124, recovery = 22).

46
Off the bus, up the stairs

Not getting any exercise because you're stuck in front of the computer all day? Did you know it's possible to exercise during the working day without even thinking about it?

Just take a moment to think about your typical workday. You get up, use the bathroom, hopefully you eat breakfast, you get the kids off to school.

You read the morning paper at breakfast or on your way to work. The bus, train or car transports you, and when you arrive perhaps you climb into the lift. You make a coffee in the staff kitchen, and then switch on your computer or whatever equipment you use. OK, so this may not exactly be your start to your workday but it's probably close enough.

Ask people why they don't exercise on workdays and the usual response is that they just don't have the time: we're working for longer hours, with greater workloads and to tighter deadlines. Now experts recommend doing 30 minutes of moderately intense physical activity on at least five days of the week to help reduce the risk of health problems such as high blood pressure. Like algebra (remember algebra?), at first glance this time and motion equation doesn't seem to work. But there are solutions.

To begin with the 30 minutes doesn't have to be all in one go. It can be 15-minute, 10-minute or even 5-minute blocks. It doesn't need to be exercise as such. It's activity that is important. Getting up and going to see a colleague rather than sending an email, going to a local coffee shop to get your mid-morning coffee rather than making it in the staff kitchen, these all count towards the 30 minutes of activity. You don't need to be sweating and panting, you just need to feel warm, slightly out of breath and for your heartbeat to increase.

So let's return to your workday routine, because this is the key, making these beneficial activities part of your routine.

At each stage of your day think about how you can change what you are doing so that you are more active doing it. For example, instead of having your morning newspaper delivered, walk to the newsagent and buy it. Perhaps you could walk with your children to school. They'll certainly benefit from this. Could you walk or cycle to work? If not, think about getting off the bus one stop earlier and walking the rest of the way. Use the stairs rather than the lift, or if you don't need the lift take a slightly longer route to your work area. Each time you have to use the stairs go up and down twice instead of just once. You'll soon feel your heart rate increasing when you do this. Rather than leaning just propping up the photocopier, walk to and from your desk while it's churning out those vital documents. Try taking a slightly longer route to the copier, and walk briskly. These all count. Amazing isn't it. In fact, by lunchtime you could have already done your 30 minutes.

Although many people seem to be able to go all day without using the bathroom, again because they are too busy, the reality is we all need to go during the day. So try this. When you need to use the bathroom, if possible use one on a different floor to the one you usually use, or use one that is further away – if you're going to do this make sure you don't wait until you're desperate! If you walk briskly there and back you could easily be achieving 25 per cent of the day's activity requirement, doing something you should be doing anyway.

You probably have meetings every now and then at work. You may have them every day. If you are having a meeting, or even just gossiping, with one or two other colleagues, rather than sitting around a table or standing still, try walking while you are talking. This is where those wearable trackers come into their own, as they can really encourage you to keep going.

47
Geeing up for the gym

However much you might hate the idea of the gym, it can prove to be extremely effective and convenient in terms of your fitness goals and it doesn't have to be boring.

When the boredom sets in it usually replaces your old friend motivation, but remember that your ultimate reward is looking and feeling sensational – it isn't meant to be a visit to a sweetshop!

Most gyms have a good range of classes ranging from yoga, Pilates, kick-boxing and circuit training to dance classes, spinning (a work-out on a stationary bike), and running and rowing clubs. Find some that suit you, and then simply enjoy them!

Which gym?

Find a gym that you'll actually go to in order to keep excuses like it not being on your way to/from work at bay. Your motto should be: Location, Location, Location!

What to do?

Most gyms will provide an induction and possibly a session with a trainer – make use of this. Decide on your goal and why you're there. Is it for weight loss, for weight gain, to train for an event, to improve fitness or to build strength? Whatever your reason, inform your trainer so they can design a programme specifically aimed at you and your needs. What about considering a personal trainer, even if you do it just once a month?

Include weight training

Weight training doesn't mean you'll end up looking like Arnie. It's a great way to add tone and definition to your body and will increase lean muscle mass, thus help to manage weight. Using weights has the added bonus of strengthening your bones. Change your technique from time to time. Challenge your body and do super-slow repetitions or try doing three or four sets back to back with just a 10-second rest in between (leave this for when you're a little more advanced).

Try these

Circuit training

This can be done in a class or you can make up your own. Keep moving from machine to machine and include free-weights and some abdominal work.

Core stability

A very important factor in overall strength, this engages the stabilising muscles and initially may feel like you're not working very hard. Take part in a class or have a trainer show you how to use the gym balls. Building up core stability can help prevent injuries and improve posture. It's a departure from just giving it welly on all the machines.

Low intensity

Include this as a great way to improve stamina and to add some variety.

Drink!

Keep yourself well-hydrated as lack of water can affect your strength, stamina and ability to burn fat.

Eat!

Don't undo all the good work with a chocolate bar after your work-out. If you're unsure about what to choose see a nutritionist.

Rest!

There is such a thing as overtraining. As you become fitter you may be able to train longer and harder, but muscles need rest to repair, recover and strengthen. Overtraining can deplete the immune system as well as your mood and energy levels.

Ouch!

If you feel pain, especially sustained pain, see someone about it – gym staff are the first port of call. Pain is the body's way of telling you something is wrong, so don't ignore it.

Look the part

Get the right kit. You'll feel like you're taking the whole thing seriously and having spent the money you'll have to turn up! Supportive, breathable shoes are a must. Find a reputable sports store that can advise you on the best shoes for your activity. Or buy online. Wear an outfit that you'll be comfortable in. You don't have to go clad in Lycra. If you feel better in shorts or jogging pants/leggings then fine, but ensure that whatever you choose allows for a good range of movement. Women: ensure that your bra offers good support for your chosen activity.

And above all ... focus!

Don't just plonk yourself on the exercise bike with your favourite weekly. Find out with the help of a trainer what your ideal training zone is. For reluctant exercisers (like me) a personal trainer can be invaluable, if expensive. With the help of my trainer I have even grown to quite like exercising. But I still hate gyms.

48
Gotta run

Run for your health, social life, waistline or sanity. There are as many reasons to run as there are runners and if you get out there and find your own perfect pace you'll never look back.

A run. A jog. A shambolic shuffle. Never mind your style or speed, the fact remains that as bipeds we were pretty much made for this running malarkey.

It's relatively cheap (though you should look to spend as much as you can afford on decent shoes and a good sports bra) and anyone can do it pretty much anywhere (though with greater and lesser degrees of pleasure). It builds up bone density, endurance, toned thighs and strengthens the heart and lungs. More than that though, for many of us it can be a special time, a quiet time set aside for thinking things over or perhaps not thinking at all.

Most runners talk about feelings of enhanced self-esteem and, while it may be tiresome to listen to, you can't help but notice the self-satisfaction, even smugness, of the hardcore harrier. Some people reach the point where if they can't run they feel out of sorts. So, what's holding you back?

For many, it's the fear that we just can't do it. So, take it one step at a time (so to speak). I know a man who found he wasn't so keen on what he saw in the mirror and so decided to try jogging. He started by running for just a few minutes, stopping to catch his breath and then running back. And he still talks of the sense of satisfaction the first time he ran over seven minutes each way – a full quarter of an hour of running. He now competes in seven-day events over hundreds of kilometres of desert.

Just take it at your own pace and plan where you will run. Take enough money to buy a bus ticket back in case you get tired or sprain something. Know where you are going and where you will find water, such as a drinking fountain, a café or from a bottle you take with you. Try not to have to cross roads (it's easy for your attention to wander at crucial moments) or run past potential stress factors such as a corner where the local kids hang out or where there's a territorial aggressive dog. Don't forget to think about the weather – runners suffer sunburn too and if there's any wind it's always easier to set out against the wind and run back with it behind you.

If you can keep going with nothing to distract you but the mirror and MTV, then good luck to you – the treadmill will be just fine. For some, however, fresh air is priority and they find it far easier to keep going when distracted by passers-by, scenery and other runners. If you feel self-conscious, try running with a mate. If you don't have a running mate then head for a park where you'll find a wide range of other joggers just like you. Perhaps even join in a parkrun or join a running club – look for adverts in your local running shop – both of which can boost your social life too. Having a running partner can make all the difference. It can make time fly as you chat, turn a fitness effort into 'quality time' with friends or family and it can help motivate you to show up in the first place. Look online and in local papers for running clubs. Many gyms also have groups of runners and they'll often be happy for newcomers to join regardless of whether or not you're a member.

Footwear

Choosing the right footwear depends on a whole host of factors such as the type of run you do, the way your foot strikes the ground as you run, the shape of your arches and your weight. Get it right and the shoe will cushion you where your foot hits the floor and help you roll across your foot and spring into the next stride. Get it wrong and in the long term you risk discomfort and even injuries. The best thing to do is to find a seriously good shoe shop (specialised running shops usually advertise themselves as such in magazines and online). Take your old shoes along with you to show them the wear pattern and never trust a salesperson who doesn't want to see you run in the shoes you try out. At least one shop I know insists on videoing your feet as you run on a treadmill and analysing your footstrike and gait. Nor does that attention to detail mean that you end up paying more. Personally I've never found specialists trying to upsell me to the latest trendy model. I can't say the same for general sports shops.

49
Have a heart (rate monitor)

Do you hate jogging/running? All that wobbly flesh jiggling up and down?

If you were to look in a mirror while out on your fit kick and see your face crunched up in agony and effort, with your tongue hanging out from the struggle of it all, you'd probably throw away your running shoes and head straight back to the couch.

Well, that's how I was until I had my Pauline conversion. You simply have to get a heart rate monitor. Now! No excuses. In my experience, this is the only way to attempt running without knackering yourself in the process. You exercise according to your own fitness level and don't try to race ahead before you're ready. Heart rate monitors are readily available online or any good sports shop; some gyms also sell them. There is a lot of wearable tech available these days but not all these devices include a true heart rate monitor (some just measure your pulse) so check before you buy.

A heart rate monitor usually has two parts: a chest strap and a sports watch. The strap picks up your heartbeat, which is displayed on the watch. In this way you can tell if your training is too strenuous or not strenuous enough. A few years back, I decided to wear my new heart rate monitor around the house while I performed a few domestic tasks. I realised my fitness needed serious attention when my heart rate, while peeling a carrot, was up through the roof!

Don't go for the all-singing, all-dancing version of the heart rate monitor to start with. There are versions that will tell you how many calories you've burned, how far you've been on your training and record all sorts of things you might want to forget. If you're new to heart rate monitors then just buy a basic model like a Polar A3. You can always trade up later if you get into it. As you can imagine, there are hundreds of models catering for various fitness audiences.

Walk the walk

Walking is a great way to get started. It's the safest work-out. We all know how to do it for starters! The intensity is low but it's great for burning fat. Walking is also a great de-stressor and doesn't require any expensive gear, just put on your heart rate monitor and a pair of trainers and hit the road. If you do decide to get into running in a serious way, you might consider an assessment with a physiotherapist who will let you know what type of stretching and other exercise would be good for you. In your hurry to get fit, it's always worth making sure that you aren't overstraining yourself in any way. A big one to watch out for is your knee health. Even taking a couple of lessons in running from a well-qualified personal trainer might save you money in the end by getting your running style right from the outset.

A heart rate monitor will:

- help you moderate your exercise intensity;

- help motivate you;

- accurately measure your heart rate; and

- enable you to judge improvement over time, like having your own personal trainer.

There are different formulae for calculating your heart rate, but presuming you're not about to train to be an Olympic sprinter go with Maffetone's 'aerobic' maximum rate, by which your optimal heart rate for aerobic training is determined by the 180 formula: your age subtracted from 180. This is fine if you've been exercising regularly (four times a week) for two years without any problems. However, if you're recovering from a major illness or on medication subtract 10 (if this applies to you, check with a doctor before you start exercising); if you've not exercised before, if exercise has been patchy, you get loads of colds or have allergies or asthma, subtract 5; if you're a competitive athlete and have been training for two years without any problems or injury, then add 5. You will then have your maximum aerobic heart rate. Your everyday training zone will then range from that number to 10 beats below that number. For example, if your maximum heartbeat is 155 then your training zone would be 145 to 155. (Thanks to Dr Philip Maffetone for this formula.) As your fitness improves, your heartbeat slows down, so you have to work harder to maintain the same heart rate.

50
Take a hike

If you're new to exercise or just don't fancy the gym, just walk away. It's easy to start, and requires no special clothing or equipment.

Most of us view walking as a way to get from A to B, and most of the time we'll choose to use the car or bus to get us to where we want to go. There is a good reason to put one foot in front of the other more often: it's a low-impact way to get fit and take in some great scenery. It is not expensive, it is not complicated and you can do it anywhere.

Half an hour's walking will help to tone up your legs and bottom. There's a catch; you won't see results with a gentle stroll to work or the shops once or twice a week. To make a difference, you'll need to walk at least three times a week, building up to five times a week, for half an hour. You'll need to do it at a reasonable pace, one that warms you up, makes you feel ever so slightly sweaty and leaves you feeling slightly breathless, but not so breathless that you could not hold a conversation. If you walk up some hills or on an incline on the treadmill in the gym, you'll increase the challenge and burn up more calories. It is simple. Here are a few other pointers to bear in mind:

You don't really need specialist gear for walking, but a decent pair of trainers will support you better than ordinary shoes. If you're planning to take up hill walking or hiking, you will need shoes or boots designed for the purpose, both for comfort and safety.

You'll work harder outdoors than inside on a treadmill as you'll have to cope with changing terrain and wind resistance. Regularly spending time outside has been shown to keep you emotionally fit, boosting feelings of well-being and staving off depression.

Wear something comfortable! It might sound obvious, but if you get wet or too hot, you'll want to give up and go back home. High-tech sports fabrics are designed to draw away sweat and protect you from wind and rain without weighing you down.

When walking, keep your tummy muscles pulled in to work your abdominal muscles and protect your back. Walk tall, avoid slumping and use your natural stride.

If you swing your arms while you walk, you'll increase your heart rate and get more of a workout.

For the best technique, hit the ground with your heel first, roll through your foot and then push off with your toes.

Rather than just randomly walking when you feel like it, try to schedule a daily walk, or at least every other day. That way, you are more likely to stick with it and see results in conjunction with your healthier eating habits, plus you'll be able to monitor your progress and feel great.

To reap the greatest benefits, set yourself a plan, say over six weeks, gradually increasing the length of time you walk and its frequency and the speed. For example, in week one you could walk for half an hour three times a week, slowly for 15 minutes and briskly for 15 minutes. Over the next few weeks, you would aim to add another walking session and making each one 5 or 10 minutes longer, and you would walk briskly for 20 or 25 minutes and at a slower pace for the rest of the time. By the end of six weeks, you could be walking for 45 minutes to an hour four or five times a week, and mostly at the faster pace.

Taking it a step further

Once you've got into walking you might find you want to organise some longer walks. For this you will need some better equipment. The gear is only necessary if you're going to take the whole thing seriously – short walks in the countryside on designated footpaths don't need full-on survival gear. But wherever you're going make sure you have a map and that you know how to read it.

Unless you live in a perpetually sunny clime some great wet-weather gear is a must. These days you can get very light wet-weather gear that will fold up and fit into your pocket. Don't just get the coat, invest in the trousers as well – you'll thank me for this one day, as there's nothing worse than being in the middle of nowhere with wet, cold and soggy trousers and no chance of changing them for the next three hours. There's no such thing as bad weather, just inappropriate gear!

The second vital bit of kit for your proper walking experience is the right boots. Get proper walking socks and try your boots on while wearing them so you don't end up with footwear that is too small. A good outdoor shop should be able to advise you on the right kind of boots and socks for you. The boots need to be protective of the ankles, waterproof and not too heavy. They also need a good grip.

The other essential piece of kit is your rucksack or daypack. Choose one with a middle strap that goes round your tummy as this will help to protect your back. These days there are rucksacks that make sure the material isn't next to your back so you don't get too sweaty carrying them. Get one with loads of pockets for maps, bits of string, etc.

Make sure you pack your rucksack with basic survival gear: matches (in a little plastic bag so they're not soggy when you need them), a Swiss army knife, foil blankets, bottles of water, oatcakes, nuts and maybe some dark chocolate (temperature permitting), and a whistle just in case you need to attract attention. A hat, good sunglasses and some sunscreen are essential on sunny days. Finally on a very long walk a small medical kit that includes some rehydration sachets (electrolyte formulas) and some plasters for those pesky blisters is a must.

Put actual dates in your diary and organise to go walking with friends. Always take water with you, however!

Take a holiday that includes guided walks in wonderful countryside. Lots of companies offer this sort of thing now: try www.atg-oxford.co.uk, which offers walks for all levels of fitness and experience. Also check out www.walksworldwide.com and www.theultimatetravelcompany.co.uk

---

51
Fancy a dip?

It's easy to turn a dip into a workout. What's more, splashing around is so much fun that it won't even feel like exercise.

Like it or not, we all know that a sedentary lifestyle does us no favours in terms of health and fitness.

Many people shy away from 'formal' exercise such as sports and the gym because they find it dull, hard to do or hard to fit into their lives. That's why I'm suggesting swimming, which most of us view as an enjoyable thing to do rather than a chore. In my experience, there seem to be very few people who really hate it. I am one of those people, but that's because I nearly drowned as a kid and wouldn't go back into the water for years – so I chose the gym over the pool every time even though I hate the gym. I now go with a friend every Friday – we swim and gossip, both of which exercise the lungs.

Swimming is great exercise, easy on your joints and lots of fun. You can even take your kids along. Just make sure that someone keeps an eye on them while you do a little more than splash about, using the following ideas.

Use different strokes to maximise the benefits

If you vary the strokes you use, you won't get bored with endless laps of front crawl. Breaststroke works on the chest muscles, shoulders, upper back, arms and thighs, while backstroke focuses on the upper back as well as the arms and stomach muscles. Crawl works the shoulders and upper back, the buttock muscles and the quads at the front of the thighs.

Try floats for extra resistance

Use a float for extra muscle toning. For the lower body, simply hold your float out in front of you and kick your legs to work your legs and bottom. If you hold the float between your legs so you can't kick them, you can concentrate on working on your arms.

Maximise your workout and feel great

Rather than swimming along at a gentle pace without getting your face wet, you'll have to get your heart rate up to really feel the benefit. One way to do this is with interval training, which means swimming fast for a length or two, then swimming more slowly. Just as you feel you're starting to recover, pick the pace up again and so on until the end of your session.

Keep it up!

As with any exercise you have to do it consistently to see results. Swim three times a week for twenty minutes as a starting point and you'll feel fitter and more toned in a month.

Breathe right

Breathing correctly stops you becoming exhausted too quickly or getting frustrated at taking in mouthfuls of water. Think of breathing for swimming in the same way as breathing when you're walking down the street. You should neither hold your breath or take in enormous gulps of air. With the crawl, for example, when you need to take a breath just turn your mouth to your right or left shoulder. When you put your head back into the water, look forward rather than down. This will help with exhalation as your windpipe is more open. Breathe out by letting the air trickle out slowly instead of blowing it out. Develop a rhythm and you'll be able to keep going for longer.

If swimming bores you but you'd like a pool workout try aqua aerobics, which is fun for just about everyone. Some exercises are done holding on to the side and others use floats. Most sessions include some sort of routine in the middle but you're never out of your depth. Try a few different classes, as instructors have different styles, and you'll like some more than others.

52
Preposterous posture

Were you always nagged to sit up straight and stop slouching? If you didn't listen, chances are you're now suffering from an even bigger pain in the neck.

Perfect posture could be your short cut to a leaner, longer shape. You'll be breathing better too. When you're hunched over, your internal organs don't have sufficient room, you don't allow enough oxygen into your body and you might also find that your digestion and circulation suffer.

Try this: Sit up straight for five minutes with your head up and shoulders dropped. Concentrate on your breathing. How do you feel? Relaxed? Of course you do! So, where can you take it next?

Pilates

Pilates may seem like a relatively new fad, but Joseph H. Pilates actually perfected his programme in the US in the 1920s. Pilates is a re-education programme for your muscles, which are used to a lifetime of abuse. It aims, through often very subtle movements, to correct these bad habits. One of the major features of Pilates is core stability and strength and one of the most difficult things to grasp is the pelvic tilt. In my opinion, you really need a teacher to take you through the basics of Pilates or you can end up wondering whether you're getting it right. Most gyms offer Pilates – take advantage of their classes because one-to-one Pilates tuition can be expensive.

Alexander technique

Think how easily small kids move. However, as we grow older and tense ourselves up against the worries of the world our posture suffers, often with disastrous results such as migraine, arthritis, neck pain and back pain. Many postural problems have stemmed from over-tensed neck muscles, which interfere with how the head relates to the spine. The Alexander Technique is often taught using verbal instruction and the physical guidance of a teacher's correcting hands. It's often taught privately so prepare yourself for an investment. Check out www.alexandertechnique. com, a comprehensive source of information.

Just be with t'ai chi

T'ai chi is a slow-moving choreography and is considered a martial art – each minute movement shifts the body's weight subtly from one leg to the other throughout the whole routine. Moment to moment attention is required at all times, thus t'ai chi is a type of meditation through movement. Practised properly, flexibility, balance and strength are all within your grasp. Think of the hundreds practising in groups in China, all silently moving in harmony – wonderful. Look for t'ai chi advertised locally. Again, many gyms now run classes. Be warned, t'ai chi is a lifelong journey, not something you master overnight.

Don't want to do the work?

What about getting a chiropractor, osteopath or physiotherapist to check your posture out and help fix it? Over time the lines between these three disciplines seem to have become a little blurred, but a chiropractor is really concerned about your spine; osteopathic treatment concentrates on the relationship between the structure of the body – the skeleton, muscles, ligaments and connective tissues – and relieving muscle tension is often a big part of the therapy; physiotherapists can assess your posture, but often make you do the work itself by giving you exercises to do at home, so this isn't so much for the lazy or undisciplined!

In my opinion you can't afford to pump it down the gym without doing these types of stretching exercises. I call it the ying and yang of exercise – you have to get the balance. Go ahead and do a pumping, thumping work-out, but feed in at least one proper posture session once a week. So, if you do three gym sessions a week, make that two plus an exercise session aimed at looking after your posture.

53

Are you sitting comfortably?

Pilates is a great way of avoiding injury and you don't have to be a dancer to benefit – the average desk jockey risks quite enough damage at work, and a few simple moves can ease the pain of the working day.

Pilates first found fame as a way for injured dancers to recover their strength and mobility. With its emphasis on building up tone with low stress and few repetitions it proved a great way of recovering dynamically – essential for those aiming to get back to full fitness as fast as possible.

These days the walking wounded that turn to it are just as likely to be office workers with back pain and stiff necks. Ironically many of them will perform their Pilates moves with great care and attention in the studio, then go back to doing exactly what caused the problem once they're back in the familiar surroundings of the office. While the studio is undoubtedly the place to learn new moves, you can practise them just about anywhere on the planet, and Pilates in the office is a great way of preventing those problems from showing up in the first place. Take it from me. I found out the hard way. A professional life slaving over a hot keyboard left me with chronic back pain, stiff hands and an amusingly lopsided neck from clutching a phone under my chin. These days I make sure I get away from the keyboard often enough to give my body a break, but when deadlines are tight, or the boss is hanging over your shoulder, you don't have to leave your seat to perform simple exercises to release those muscles, help your posture and above all ease the stress.

Pilates at the keyboard

Sitting isn't as easy as it looks. In fact done incorrectly it is so bad for us that I think of it as the new smoking. Standing desks and walking meetings are taking off in some trendy companies but most of us will end up sitting at a desk for much of our working lives. We manage to put stress on our shoulders, necks and backs just by the way we sit. Pilates posture can help.

First, make sure you're sitting back in your chair with your feet flat on the floor. Imagine that your coccyx (tailbone) is made of lead and pulling straight down into the chair. Make sure your spine is in neutral and you can feel the middle of your back lightly pressed against the seat back. Your shoulders should be relaxed but not slumped, and your stomach tucked in. To get a feel for that position try some leg lifts. Lift each knee alternately up, placing it smoothly down again with the foot flat on the floor. You should be totally stable, if you can feel your coccyx moving, then check that you are sitting back and in the neutral position – you may be sitting too far forward with your pelvis tilted. If you're unsure whether you are sitting neutrally, then try lifting the knee right up towards your chest. As you do you'll reach a point where you can feel the pelvis tilt, and the coccyx slides towards the front of the seat. Hopefully that feel for being out of neutral should help you settle into neutral.

With your pelvis and back sorted out, the next issue is your shoulders and the neck strain that all too easily results from tension and poor posture. Hunching your shoulders upwards is a shortcut to tension and trouble as it tightens the trapezius muscle at the top of your back and that transmits its strain into the back of the neck. If you feel tense (and who doesn't at some point in the working day) then try this.

Slide your shoulder blades towards each other and then down and at the same time extend your neck. You should feel an immediate easing of the pressure on your spinal column, shoulders and neck as well as feeling as if you've just grown an inch. Next time you want to shout at someone, try doing that first.

A really great time to try sitting exercises is on the bus/tube or at the traffic lights on the way home. Because we're tired we're likely to slump and take all that tension back home with us. Try and make it part of your daily routine to ease that pressure out as a way of leaving work behind before you get home. Don't forget that it's just as effective in the pub or sat in front of your favourite TV programme.

The lift is another exercise you can do at your office chair or on the bus. The aim is to work on zipping up from the bottom of the pelvis towards your ribs. While sitting upright, imagine that there is a lift on your pelvic floor. As you breathe out try to take that lift 'up' to the next floor – you should feel your pelvic muscles go taut. As you take the 'lift' further up the floors from 'first' to 'second', you should feel your lower abdominals tighten. Higher than that and you risk the six-pack muscling in on the action.

Unrolling the stress

Since we tend to store up stress in the shoulders, try to roll it out again with shoulder rotations. Your shoulder is a ball and socket joint, meaning it can rotate in any direction, so every now and again you should let it. Sitting in neutral, with your feet flat on the floor and your shoulders relaxed but not slumped, bend your elbows and rest your fingertips on your shoulder (right on right, left on left). Now circle them forwards and upwards so your elbows touch, then lift up above your ears, pull back to be in line with your shoulders and finally come forward again. Now perform the same circle but in the opposite direction – remember the importance of working every equal and opposite muscle so that for every pull there is a push.

The best office de-stressing exercise is undoubtedly to land a clean right hook on the boss, but since this may lead to ugliness it's worth looking at other options.

Stress balls – those squidgy balls you can squash in your fist when anxiety rises – are a good exercise for your hand muscles. The problem is people often tense the trapezius muscle that leads to the shoulders when they do. If you use a stress ball, make sure you perform the shoulder roll above after you've used it.

Now work on the fingers – if you've been typing, then they're probably tense and tired. Despite the publicity about RSI you only have to look around any office for a couple of minutes and you'll find keyboards without wrist wrests, keyboards set up at the wrong height for the seat and keyboards right at the edge of the desk so there's nowhere to rest your elbows. Concentrated mouse work, even with elegantly shaped ergonomic mice, can also put real pressure on your fingers.

To release tension in the fingers start by turning your hands palm upwards and bring the tip of each finger in turn to the tip of your thumb then repeat the sequence. Just to make things a little more interesting, try starting with the little finger on one hand at the same time as you start at the index finger on the other so the two hands are out of synch.

Next, hold all your fingers out flat together and then open up the gap between the second and third fingers so that the first and second pull away in one direction and the third and fourth in the other. Sci-fi fans will immediately recognise this as the Vulcan greeting. Now bring the second and third fingers together and keep them together and this time open up the gaps between the first and second, and third and fourth. Try not to do this if the self-appointed office wit is around, otherwise Spock/Mork and Mindy gags will follow you around forever.

Put your arm up in the air, bend your elbow and allow your hand to rest on the top of your head with your fingers on the side just touching your ear. Now gently ease into a stretch by pulling very lightly with the hand while resisting gently with the head and neck muscles as if you were trying to straighten your neck against the pull of your hand. Don't overdo it: this is a gentle release of the muscles in the neck for just a few seconds. Now reverse arms and do the other side. Now roll your head back and circle.

There, feel slightly less homicidal now?

54

Stand tall, breathe deep

It takes five times as much energy to slouch as it does to stand straight. If you aren't standing properly, your body has to work harder.

The very simplest step for boosting energy is to ensure your posture is tiptop. This ensures you are breathing well, which means oxygenation of the tissues is maximised.

But there's more to it than that – the effects of standing tall have a profoundly energising effect on our psyche. Once I interviewed a consultant radiologist whose speciality was osteoporosis – the thinning of the bones that, in extreme cases, causes a hump so that the sufferer has no choice but to stare downwards. He was almost moved to tears by his patients' fate. 'Can you imagine the indignity of living like that, face down, slumped forward, unable to meet anyone's eye?' he told me. 'The pain my patients go through is bad enough, but the effect on their spirits is worse.'

What amazes me is that so many of us (myself included) do that to ourselves willingly. Neuro-linguistic programming – a highly successful form of mind coaching – teaches that changing the body's posture improves mood immediately. Start with these simple changes and see if it doesn't improve your view of the world.

Standing – get neutral

Stand with your weight balanced equally between your two feet.

Make your knees soft and pull yourself up gently through your thighs, your hips, your spine. Relax your shoulders and let them fall away from your ears.

Now check your pelvis position. Place the heels of your hands on your hip bones and position your fingertips so they are pointed downwards towards your pubic bone. Now adjust your pelvic position so the heels of your hands are on the same plane as your fingers, with your fingertips neither in front of nor behind the heels of your hands. You may have to contract your abdominals so that your navel goes nearer to your spine.

Sitting – the rule of 90

When you are sitting in a chair, as often as possible observe the rule of 90. This means that your back is at 90 degrees to your thighs thus preventing slumping or leaning forward. A lumbar cushion at the base of the back of the chair behind your coccyx is worth investing in if you work for a lot of the time in a seated position. Or roll up a towel and use this instead.

Your calves should form a 90-degree angle with your thighs at the knee. You may have to use a stool to raise your feet.

Spine stretcher

This is a great exercise for freeing up your spine when you have been forced to maintain the same position for too long. It also gives you the advantages of an 'inversion exercise' – blood flowing to the brain – which wakes you up.

Stand against a wall with every bit of your spine against the wall. Now starting from the top, the neck, peel your spine off the wall, vertebra by vertebra. Move slowly breathing easily until your lumbar (lower) vertebrae are off the wall and you are hanging forward with your hands reaching towards the ground. Feel the pull of gravity in your spine as your head hangs downwards. Now slowly reposition your spine against the wall, moving upwards, with the lumbar spine reaching the wall first.

Walk the plank

Good posture is easy when you have a strong band of muscles around your middle – like a corset, your back and stomach muscles hold your body upright. This exercise is called the plank and it's a favourite of personal trainers because it increases your 'core strength' – which is just what you need to stand tall, breathe deeply and thus have more energy.

- Lie face down on the floor with your hands next to your shoulders.

- Lift yourself onto your hands as if you were about to do a press up, and on your toes so that your back is straight. Your neck should form a line with your spine and your face look towards the floor.

- Pull in your stomach muscles. Your spine should be flat, resembling a plank.

Tough, isn't it? But if you can do it, you'll stand taller than ever. On your first attempt, if you can manage this properly for thirty seconds, you're doing well. Build up from there to a couple of minutes daily. And it helps to have a friend check out that you are doing it properly, i.e. your back is straight. Remember it's called the plank because that's what you should resemble: if your back sags, you could injure yourself.

55
Stretching the point

Stretching is one of those things we know we should do, don't really know why and quietly forget about when no one's looking.

If you've decided to become more active you'll be using your muscles more intensively and taking them through a greater range of movement. Fail to stretch and you'll recover more slowly from your efforts, be stiffer, run the risk of injury and, worse, end up walking like John Wayne.

Pre-stretches

These prepare your body for what's to come. There's a lot of argument about this since many people, including myself, think you run more risk of damaging yourself by stretching when cold than actually doing any good. Similarly, while many gyms offer a 'stretching' class, very few will make sure you warm up properly beforehand. So, if you're going to do a stretching class then make sure you warm up thoroughly (jog, row, cycle) so that the appropriate areas are really ready to rumble.

Maintenance stretch

This is done at the end of your exercise or during it in the form of stretch breaks (very handy for a sneaky excuse to catch your breath). The aim of maintenance stretching is to help your muscles resume their normal length after working harder. You should hold the stretch for just 10 to 15 seconds or so. Remember to stretch all of the muscles you're using – for example, new runners often remember to stretch their legs, but forget the hip flexors at the top of the pelvis that are used to raise the knee in the direction of the chest.

Developmental stretching

This is all about trying to stretch the muscles further and longer so they become more flexible and better at your chosen activity. Start stretching as normal and hold the stretch for 8–10 seconds while your muscle relaxes into the new position. Then go further into the stretch and continue the count up to 20 seconds to complete the stretch.

Common stretches

There's a stretch for every part of your body, including a few you're probably not familiar with yet. Take time to find out about the stretches specific to your sport and then take the time to do them. The most common stretches are:

Quadriceps

While standing upright, balance on one leg and bend the other so you can catch your foot in your hand. Flex your foot gently back up to your buttocks and don't worry about putting a hand out on a wall or partner to keep your balance. Very slightly bend the knee of the leg you're balancing on and tip the hips forward to feel the stretch down the front of your thigh. Hold. Gently go back to standing and switch legs.

Calves

Stand four or five steps away from and facing a wall. Keep your left foot in its original position but place your right foot halfway between you and the wall. Reach forward with your outstretched arms so you're leaning against the wall with them. Your right leg should now be bent and your left leg straight out behind you with the sole of the foot flat on the floor. Feel the stretch up the back of the calf. Hold, then gently go back to standing and switch legs.

Triceps

Reach one arm straight up above your head then bend it at the elbow so your hand is now behind your neck. Reach up with the other hand, take the first elbow, and gently pull it down and across in the direction of the pulling arm's shoulder. Hold, release, switch.

Shoulder

Hold your arm out straight in front of you then move it across your body placing the other hand on the upper arm between elbow and shoulder. Use that hand to push the arm in towards the chest. Hold, release, switch.

Never go into a stretch to the point where it hurts. You should feel the stretching, but actual pain is never a good thing. Gently build the stretch up little by little over a matter of weeks until you can get to the point where you stretch that far without hurting. And don't bounce into your stretches – professional athletes in explosive sports like jumping and sprinting use so-called 'ballistic' stretches, but for the rest of us it's just an invitation to injury.

If you like the idea of developmental stretching and would like to be suppler, try Bikram yoga. Sessions are conducted in a steamy room to keep muscle temperatures high and help suppleness. There's only one set of moves so it's easy to learn but takes forever to master. The emphasis is on developing the range of movement and stretch in joints and muscles.

56
Yoga

Yoga is about being rather than doing. It's non-competitive and a great balancer for the type of exercise you might do at the gym.

Not so long ago, if you admitted you did yoga you'd have been classed as a New Age weirdo and given a wide berth. Today, if you're not into yoga you're the weird one. So, get with the programme!

Although yoga has evolved to incorporate quite a few different types, you're missing the point if you're using yoga to 'get a work-out'. Check out www.yogapoint.com for a guide to all the different types of yoga and pick the one that sounds interesting for you. You might want to experiment with the different types by going to a few classes. Or ask around, as friends might be able to give you advice.

In essence though, all types of yoga are about using the body and breathing to help calm the mind in order to produce a feeling of well-being. Yoga is a great stress buster if ever there was one and it's easy to do at any age so it's never too late to start. Flexibility is a vital component, both physically and mentally – a flexible mind equals a flexible body. Yoga generally uses asanas (postures) that usually retain their ancient names: the fish, the bridge, the bow, the scorpion, etc. They are believed to bring benefits to different areas of the body and are held for a period of time to stretch and strengthen muscles. The shoulder-stand asana, for example, is said to massage the thyroid and bring benefits to the mind through improving blood circulation to the head. Worth a try? The simplest asana is the corpse position, which involves lying down on your back on the floor with your eyes closed. Your breathing should be slow and steady, and your arms should be held at a 45-degree angle away from the body (not an excuse for a kip though, apparently).

Yoga is really a lifestyle rather than simply an exercise discipline. It incorporates 'proper' breathing or relaxation and a 'proper' diet. It's powerful stuff that's deceptively simple and amazingly dynamic. A proper diet, according to the yogis, is usually a vegetarian diet comprising Sattvic foods such as wholemeal grains and fresh fruit and vegetables. Diet as a whole is divided up into three main sections: Sattvic foods, which I've already mentioned; Rajasic foods, which are hot and bitter foods (e.g. coffee, tea, chocolate, salt, strong herbs, fish) that are considered to destroy the mind–body equilibrium; and Tamasic foods (e.g. meat, alcohol, garlic, onions), which benefit neither mind nor body as they encourage a sense of inertia. Stale or unripe food is also considered Tamasic.

As an alternative to hiring a private teacher, which can be quite expensive, club together with a couple of friends for some really worthwhile tuition in a small group once a week. You can always go to classes at the gym the rest of the time.

57
Breathe in, breathe out!

Proper breathing can be a forgotten art for people in stressful jobs, lives or relationships. And these days we often hold onto our breath out of sheer terror.

It's not called the life breath for nothing. With each breath we exchange carbon dioxide from inside the body with life-giving oxygen from outside. If this incredible process was interrupted for more than a few minutes, it would be curtains.

The partner to breathing is an amazingly reliable muscle: your heart. Oxygen-rich blood is pumped by the heart from the lungs via the arteries and small capillaries to all the cells of the body. This allows the cells to function. Carbon dioxide is then transported back to the heart through the veins and from there it's pumped to the lungs and we breathe it out. The whole process starts again with our next in-breath. Breathing is an amazing, miraculous process and it's worked so well that it hasn't changed one iota since we were running away from sabre-toothed beasties. Sometimes, however, that's just the problem.

We may think that we're civilised humans who know the difference between Armani and Asda, but the fact is that as far as our ancient intuitive response mechanisms go, we're just another animal fighting for our tiny space in the (concrete) jungle. We humans go through the same physiological reaction as a cat does when it's dumped in a barrel of freezing water or being chased by a dog, or as a mouse does when a cat is stalking it for that matter.

When faced with what we perceive as a danger (this could be your tax bill, your boss or being late for work), we go into a state of hyperarousal known as the flight-or-fight response. You might think that hyperarousal sounds a bit saucy, but it actually means feelings like anxiety, rage or sheer blind terror. The resulting flight-or-fight mechanism is unbelievably clever and causes a rapid cascade of nervous-system firings and the release of powerful hormones like adrenaline. We become hyperaware of all our surroundings, the pupils of our eyes dilate to let in more light, the hair on our body stands up so that we become more sensitive to vibrations, the digestive system shuts down and the heart rate shoots up so that there's more blood available for legging it up a tree at top speed. And that's just for starters! Here's the technical part – you've just activated the sympathetic part of your autonomic nervous system. Impress your friends with that one!

This brings us back to breathing. Breathing centres you. It's almost impossible to be stressed if breathing is measured, calm and deep. Breathing overrides the powerful stress response and slows down the reaction of the autonomic nervous system. So, the good news is that you have some degree of control over how you react to stress.

Breathing exercises

Breathing exercises are deceptively simple and dynamically powerful. All you need is a few minutes a day to provide you with a powerful way of dealing with stress. There are hundreds of different exercises you could do. I'm going to give you just two for starters. Do them! Don't just read this and think it's for someone else. It's for you. It's for us all!

Exercise 1: observing the breath

Sit on a comfortable chair, making sure that your feet are on the ground. Close your eyes, rest one hand in your lap and place the other on your tummy. You should feel the tummy expanding as you breathe in and contracting as you breathe out. Breathe in deeply through your nose and silently count 'one'. Breathe out. Breathe in again and count 'two'. Do this for up to 10 breaths and then do it the other way round. Breathe in. Breathe out and count 'one'. Breathe in. Breathe out and count 'two'. Do this for five rounds to start with, building up to 10. Do this once a day.

Exercise 2: anti-stress breath

Try this if you find yourself stressed out and in need of some immediate relief. Breathe in for four counts, hold for four counts and exhale for four counts. Remember to let the out-breath out slowly, not in a rush. Do this for about five cycles, being careful that you don't overdo it otherwise you could end up feeling a bit dizzy.

Put the breathing exercises in your diary initially and write reminders on sticky notes on your bathroom mirror. It takes around 21 days to form a habit, but once you're into it, the habit will stick.

Part 4

Wellness – it's all in the mind

58

The way we're working isn't working

(with apologies to Tony Schwartz)

I think that this is a great title for a book and I wish I had thought of it first. If you want a more detailed take on this subject I can wholeheartedly recommend Schwartz's book as a very enlightening read. For this chapter I have grabbed a few of his themes, had a think about them and added my take. So my views don't necessarily represent his – hence the apologies!

I love Tony's observation that the 'defining ethic in the modern workplace is more, bigger, faster. More information than ever is available to us, and the speed of every transaction has increased exponentially, prompting a sense of permanent urgency and endless distraction. We have more emails to answer, more phone calls to return, more tasks to juggle, more meetings to attend, more places to go and more hours we feel we must work to avoid falling further behind.' As Gandhi was once meant to have said, 'There is more to life than simply increasing its speed.' This has never resonated more than it does today, but speed has been a driving force for humanity since some bright spark invented the wheel.

My feeling is that the whole way we are working, the very structure, isn't one that supports well-being in the first place. From the standard 9 to 5 day, to the relentless drive to get things done and achieve we are working outside our natural rhythms, becoming cogs in the machine. And to what purpose? Acccording to Schwartz a huge number of us are dissatisfied with our work because the relationship of the employer buying employee hours for money is a one-dimensional relationship which does not allow for the very nature of being human. Besides having sufficient money to live on, we need a lot of other basic physical, emotional, mental and spiritual needs to be met in order to be happy, fulfilled and productive. We are human beings but have become human doings. A new way of working would entail re-engagement with our bodily self, not only to earn money for our families, but being satisfied and fulfilled, dare we say happy, whatever our role. Meeting our physical, emotional, mental and spiritual needs, lets us fulfil our corresponding needs, says Schwartz – sustainability, security, self-expression, and significance, and we build our capacity to generate more and more value over time.

Physical needs

Obviously we were designed to move, yet many of us are trapped at our desks, hunched over a keyboard – endlessly forwarding more facts to someone else for processing. The physical is not just about getting out of work at the end of the day and pounding it at the gym for an hour by way of compensation. It is about movement. And keeping moving.

The new trend is for standing desks – is this something you could see working at your workplace? If not, just getting up and moving around helps, as does making sure you are sitting correctly when you are at your desk. Your workplace may have somebody to assess the ergonomic appropriateness of your desk. If not, you will have to try improve your posture by adjusting your chair and computer in a way that is comfortable for you. Chapter 52 has more on this, while Chapter 53 contains some ideas for exercises to do at your desk. Once you lose your ability to move well, it can really interfere with your well-being from both a physical and spiritual angle. Just take a look at older friends and relatives: they may be sharp as tacks mentally but if they don't have their physical movement and strength they are curtailed in all aspects of their life.

'Physical needs' means taking care of your nutrition too. Obviously you (and certainly I) can't be perfect all the time, but the real rule on this one is the one I bang on about throughout the book: Eat Real Food. Accelerate this to the top of your priority list and invest the time it needs to achieve your nutrition makeover. If you are so busy you can't do this then maybe, just maybe you need to assess if your job is working for you.

Emotional needs

The workplace often doesn't let us harness and develop our strengths as emotional beings. Often it is how we perceive ourselves to be treated by our line manager and our colleagues that determine how we feel about the job. It is said that people join companies and leave line managers. Quite often small things such as a thank you, said and meant, can go a long way to motivating us. It is time that companies really appreciated us as these emotional human beings. If you are a manager think about how you can nurture this side of your people and if you are the one being managed, consider how you might change your work habits to draw that thank you out of your line manager. If that is not going to happen, it's a question of changing how you react to your environment and the people in it or giving some serious thought to finding a new workplace.

Mental needs

Many companies push staff beyond what is reasonable for the human mind to deal with (in terms of stress and pressure), but recently mindfulness training has gone a long way to help companies train their people to become more focused and strategically driven, and less reactive to tasks and situations. Nurturing our most important asset, our mind, is one of the keys to better performance and happiness at work.

Spiritual needs

This is a 'flakey' no-no word for a lot of companies – but it simply means helping people develop shared values and purpose, and fostering respect in the workplace. Companies run like this, rather than those where the ego-driven predator, the territorial alpha ape is valued, are much beter places to work.

How can you work better?

- Physical – get moving, get up from your desk, take breaks, walk. Eat Real Food. Don't fear fat: good fats in foods such as avocados and small, oily fish such as sardines, pilchards and herring.

- Emotional – understand your mind so that you can operate in the calm, optimistic, challenged, engaged and invigorated zone, which produces sensations such as being carefree, peaceful, mellow and positive. Staying in the exhausted, depressed, sad and hopeless quadrant makes you feel reactive and negative. In the short term work towards improving your boundaries at work. How can you ensure that you leave work at a reasonable time, and that when you do that time is yours for doing the things you love, be it base-jumping, bell-ringing or flower-arranging?

- Mental – could mindfulness help? It is great to improve focus – a mental work-out. I walk and try and be present, I bring my mind back to the present when it wanders. I try not to focus on bad news but bring myself back to how I feel. Noticing feelings, both 'good' and 'bad', *is* being mindful. For more on this see Chapters 59 and 60, and Mark Williams' book, *Mindfulness*).

- Spiritual – developing compassion both for yourself and others helps and can be a good place to start in terms of gaining perspective on your values and behaviours. While the meaning of 'spiritual' is highly subjective, being the best we can be in all senses is probably something that we know how to be in our heart of hearts, and even having intention to be that person is a good start.

- Read *The way we're working isn't working* by Tony Schwartz. While you are at it read *The chimp paradox* by Professor Steve Peters – this book is a must for anyone trying to understand their own mind and behaviour as well as everyone else's.

59
Using Mindfulness at work[*]

What is Mindfulness?

Mindfulness is a way of being more aware of everything that we are experiencing, in the here and now, that helps us not only enjoy life more but also be better at everything we do.

Being mindful means using the more cognitive areas of the brain to experience greater clarity about everything that is going on around us as well as the stories that our minds are telling us.

There are formal Mindfulness practices, which are very effective and well worth learning, such as a Body Scan (scanning your body, area by area, with focused attention on what sensations you are aware of in each area) or Breathing practice (focused attention to the sensations of the breath in the body). These Mindfulness practices are as beneficial for the mind as exercise is for the muscles of the body. Just as the body becomes fit through taking exercise, so a person becomes more mindful by practising Mindfulness exercises daily. (Mindfulness at Work has short practises on its website that you can download, including a free three-minute breathing practise.)

But being Mindful is something that you aim to be, as much as you can during your day, not just for the 10 minutes you might be practising your Body Scan. It's a way of life – or rather a way of approaching life.

[*] Thanks to Mindfulness at Work Ltd (www.Mindfulnessatwork.com) for Chapters 59 and 60

By being more mindful, we learn to observe thoughts as just thoughts, acknowledging that they are not necessarily facts. We learn to become the witness to the emotions that these thoughts can trigger, and the reactions in the body that can also result. We look to acknowledge these thoughts, emotions and sensations with a compassionate objectivity which enables us to see them for what they are, without judging them. This enables us to come off autopilot and learn to respond rather than react to life – making wiser choices and feeling calmer in the process.

Why Mindfulness at work?

Because Mindfulness helps us be better at lots of different workplace activities – from sustaining focused attention for long periods and problem solving, to getting on better with our colleagues and having more emotional and physical resilience. People who practise Mindfulness techniques for just 10 minutes a day have been shown to have increased the grey matter in their pre-frontal cortex after just 4 weeks of training – giving them greater 'executive' functioning and a more positive attitude. They have also altered the neural pathways in their brain – so instead of having the amygdala (which controls the brain's fight-or-flight response) hijack the mind and elicit a reactionary response to a potentially stressful situation at work, a more considered response brought about by using the more advanced areas of the brain can take place. This can be so helpful when decisions need to be made quickly or a colleague's behaviour appears threatening. It means that a more objective, considered and less emotional response can occur and this is better for everyone involved. Mindfulness helps people see things from another's point of view – by teaching Beginner's Mind – enabling more effective conflict resolution and greater creativity too. The practice of Mindfulness is a time-tested antidote to operating on autopilot. Research at Duke University demonstrates why. It was discovered that more than forty per cent of our actions are based on habits, not conscious decisions.

Certain unconscious habits and assumptions seem to have become hard-wired in us, but if we bring them into focus the force of these habits will no longer determine our behaviour and the outcome of certain aspects of our lives.

And with greater working memory and increased cortical folding (more folding equals greater cortex surface area and therefore more brain power) reversing the ageing process and the increase in antibodies delivering improved immunity, Mindfulness not only helps people to get better at their jobs but gives them the resilience to sustain their role effectively.

Mindfulness-based stress reduction therapy (MBSR) has been shown to reduce anxiety in a broad range of people, as reported by the University of Ottawa. Mindfulness reduces stress and enhances forgiveness, according to a study published by the *Journal of American College Health*. And Mindfulness practitioners have a greater ability to moderate the intensity of their emotional arousal during stressful situations, say the Russian Academy of Medical Sciences.

Studies have shown that practising Mindfulness increases our brain's levels of GABA, DHEA, melatonin, serotonin, HGH and endorphins, making us feel much better. And Mindfulness reduces our levels of the stress hormone cortisol – which is responsible for trunkal obesity, increased glucose levels leading to Type 2 diabetes and the elevated hormone levels that can cause heart disease. Additionally, Mindfulness lowers your blood pressure, according to research published by the National Institute of Mental Health.

Mindfulness teaches us that there are several lenses through which we can look at all life experiences. Mindfulness at Work calls these The 7 Circles of Being™. Any problem can be worked through using these seven attitudes, starting with being aware of the judging and non-judging that might be taking place with regard to a given situation. By trying to approach the subject without judgement, with Patience and then Beginner's Mind, it's possible to bring different information and thoughts into view.

By applying Trust to your increased awareness and then trying to sit with it in a Non-Striving way, Accepting the situation as it is (because without acknowledging where you really are, it's difficult to chart an accurate course to where you would like to be) and then Letting Go of preconceptions, then it is remarkable what epiphanies can occur and what outcomes can be achieved.

And whether we are suffering from iterative thinking in the middle of the night which is stopping us from getting a good night's sleep, are mindlessly overeating, are not enjoying the fruits of our labours by noticing the beauty that is often under our noses or seem to be succumbing to every bug going round the office, Mindfulness can help.

Lack of sleep

Through practising Mindfulness techniques, when we become aware of how our mind can randomly jump from thought to thought, like a monkey jumping from branch to branch through the forest, we learn to smile inwardly to ourselves, gently bring our mind back from its ramblings and place its attention on the breath – focusing on the breath quietly coming in and out of the body. Ruminating on a tricky situation is unlikely to bring a solution at three o'clock in the morning (and if it does, we are even less likely to remember it later), so by focusing on our breath we quieten the mind and experience respite from the anxious thoughts and the corresponding emotions and bodily sensations that these thoughts can trigger.

Overeating

By practising mindful eating (being aware of every mouthful that we take, acknowledging everything that our senses are experiencing) we can enjoy our food more and, paradoxically, end up eating less.

The next chapter provides an exercise that will help you take the first steps towards more mindful living.

60
Raisin your awareness

Try the raisin awareness experiment, which will help you experience both Mindful Eating and Beginner's Mind.

Take one raisin and place it in the palm of your hand, imagining that you have never seen this object before and do not have a name for it.

Holding

Allow the object to rest in the palm of your hand.

Become aware of its weight.

See if you can discern its temperature.

Looking

Really look at the object, giving it your full attention.

What do you see?

Perhaps noticing its colour, shape and sheen.

Touching

Be aware of the movement as you pick the object up between thumb and forefinger of your other hand.

How does the outside texture of the object feel as you roll it gently between these fingers.

Squeezing it gently, notice what happens now: is there a sense of its interior texture?

Notice how you are feeling both the exterior and the interior textures.

Seeing

Now lift the object to a comfortable height where you can focus on it and really examine it in much more detail.

Notice its highlights and shadows and how these may change as the light catches it.

See if you can discern the object as if you're examining the contours and plains of a valley.

Hearing

Bring the object to your ear, noticing again the movement of your arm and head as you do so.

As you continue to squeeze the object gently between your fingers, are there any sounds you can hear?

Smelling

Now begin to move the object towards your mouth, again noticing the movement of your muscles.

Bring it up to your nose and notice its fragrance, really exploring this and noting any words or images that come to mind.

Are there any changes underway in your mouth or stomach?

Placing

Bring the object to your lips. Briefly explore the delicate sensation of touch here.

Place the object in your mouth without chewing, and let it rest on your tongue, noticing any sensations here.

Be aware of whether it makes any contact with the roof of your mouth.

Slowly move the object to your back teeth, being aware of the movement of muscles engaged here.

As you place the object between the teeth, are there any impulses here?

Tasting

Take a single bite and notice any sensations. Are there flavours and any other senses?

Take another bite and see what this brings.

Then another bite and so on, each time being open to what comes.

Chewing

Slowly, very slowly, chew the raisin.

Are there any sounds, sensations of texture, of flavour?

Keep chewing slowly in this way until there is almost nothing left to chew.

Swallowing

When there is almost nothing left to chew, swallow and see if you can be aware of the very intention to swallow even before the action arises.

Are you aware of the bits as they move down your throat?

Awareness

How do you feel now that you've completed the exercise?

Make a list of different ways you can become more aware of your 'here and now' experience, so that next time you are enjoying a meal, your mind isn't already transporting you to the washing-up that needs to be done, the bins that need to go out or the difficult meeting you might (or might not) have tomorrow. It's amazing how much we miss of life when we aren't being Mindful.*

---

*   There are many courses out there that can teach you the basics. Mindfulness at Work Ltd teaches short introductory courses in the workplace – they are easy to access and very powerful. Visit their website www. Mindfulnessatwork.com for further details or ask your HR department if they are planning any Mindfulness training for employees any time soon.

61
The art of doing nothing

Some days it's best to just stay under your duvet. Try to convince your family to move in with you and make a teepee of fun for the day. Retreating from the world is a restorative and something you should definitely do as regularly as you can.

We're funny creatures, aren't we? We get two weeks' holiday maybe twice a year and we try and fill it with as much as humanly possible. Yet the most relaxing holiday I've ever had was right here at home when I was waiting on a contract for something and so couldn't leave the country. I spent most of the week reading in bed, like I used to do as a child.

Someone once said, 'We are human beings, not human doings' and, you know, whoever it was is quite right. Sometimes you just need to be rather than do. Being can involve contemplation or it can involve nothing more exerting than just vegging out and grunting in response to others for a day or so.

You can't continuously behave in this way as then you'd be a person apart from society and, well, you'd probably be wanting to find yourself a mountain somewhere rather than read books on inner peace. However, you can occasionally opt out of it all. You can say, 'I'm not going to work. I'm not getting dressed. I'm not doing anything.' In the States, they have a very honest concept called 'duvet days'; here in the UK, we have the time-honoured tradition of the 'sickie'. I'm not advocating lying to the people who pay your wages, merely negotiate a duvet day with your boss (perhaps a day off in lieu of weekend or overtime work?).

Also think about all the non-work things you do: the shopping, the housework, the helping with homework, the personal grooming, the buying of presents, the social engagements, the dinner parties and the weekend breaks. Are you exhausted yet? I'm feeling like I need a lie-down just looking at that list. We seem to be hell-bent on filling every single moment of time with something useful. If we're not doing all that then we're on the computer, emailing friends that we haven't seen in ages. And why haven't we seen them? Because we're too busy!

Then when we do get around to seeing our friends, we feel compelled to have interesting things to tell them about so we run to the latest exhibition or to see a movie and a lot of it is geared towards remaining 'current' rather than true enjoyment. And so it goes on and on.

I remember a saner time. A time when, as a child, there was nothing to do so we just hung out. We'd walk down to the park or we'd go and collect conkers in the churchyard or we'd just sit on a wall and wait for the ice cream van. I'm the last person to hark back to a nostalgic, bygone era but I do think we've lost the art of doing nothing much in particular.

If you're a particularly social person, try a month of accepting no invitations. No parties, cinema trips, dinners or sports dates. And don't invite anyone to yours either. A whole month of abstinence will make you realise how much leisure time you actually have and you can then use it wisely after your month's fast to choose just those activities that truly make you happy rather than those you do out of a sense of obligation.

62

Because you're worth it

Feeling down in the dumps with nothing to look forward to? In need of something to put a smile on your face? Some self-indulgent me-time always comes up trumps.

If your get up and go has got up and gone, this idea will give you the strength to go after it.

Feeling worse for wear? A little pampering and preening can be incredibly revitalising, raising your mood, confidence and self-esteem.

Rise and shine

Waking up early and can't get back to sleep? Instead of lying there worrying, injecting a little effort into your morning routine will bring day-long benefits. Looking chic and sophisticated compared to dull and dreary makes a whopping difference to how people treat you and how you feel. Not convinced? How would you feel in response to these two statements?

'You look really tired. Are you OK?'

'Wow, you look amazing. Love the new suit.'

It might sound obvious but wearing vibrant colours will give you more zip and zing than dressing in drab browns or greys.

If you're strapped for cash right now, then perhaps it's time to check out some charity shops. You should be able to inject some pizzazz into your wardrobe on the cheap (and a fashion mistake that hasn't crippled your credit card is much easier to live with!). If the second-hand pickings are slim where you live, then give eBay a whirl: there's lots of interesting clothing to be had out there in cyberspace.

Make up your mind

Putting on make-up might be the last thing you feel like doing when you're depressed, but the old saying 'outer beauty, inner strength' has a lot of truth in it. Ever wondered why your granny called it war paint? Researchers investigated the effects of make-up on our moods by giving daily makeovers to elderly people suffering from incontinence. Three months into the experiment, a third of the elderly were out of their incontinence pads. Make-up helped them recover their dignity and sense of worth.

Many hospitals employ beauticians to improve the well-being of cancer patients. Most psychiatric departments are sadly lagging behind. I once came across a hospital ward where one of the nurses ran a weekly 'beauty group'. She styled people's hair, did mini manicures and generally made people look and feel a million dollars. It convinced me that the trusty lipstick and mascara combo can transform the way you feel. Treating yourself to some new vibrant eye colours might seem like just an instant pick-me-up, but it also gives you a little confidence boost every time you use them.

Hair's an idea for you

Are perms the new Prozac? Probably not, but if you're fed up or feeling fusty, half an hour at your hairdresser is great for hauling up your humour. Many hairdressers have first-rate listening skills. The best have the sort of interested empathy many shrinks can only dream of, and a humble cut and blow dry can turn into an impromptu therapy session. With the right stylist even when you go in dejected and dishevelled you'll come out sleek, sexy and smiling. The lift you get might not last longer than your retouched roots, but it could become the highlight of your month.

Look good, feel great

Tense and on edge? Unwind and rejuvenate at a beauty parlour or day spa. While a bikini wax may well make you cry, a hot stone massage, age-defying facial or airbrush tan are sure to make you feel like one of the happy people. Even if only for a couple of hours. Guys, no need to be shy. Take your pick from wet shaves, sports massage and other indulgences from the male spruce-up menu.

Believe in yourself

Self-belief is a vital human attribute that most of us take for granted until it deserts us. It is the 'wind beneath our wings' that contributes significantly to our state of well-being, enabling us to perform under pressure and duress. A few possess a demi-godlike level of self-belief that appears to banish all self-doubt. For most of us mortals, we have to work at keeping faith in ourselves. It is vital for our mental health that we work at bolstering our self-belief. Lowered self-esteem and confidence has been shown to be implicated in a range of adjustment difficulties (e.g. truancy and gang membership) and mental health problems (e.g. eating disorders, depression).

Helpfully, two researchers (Ralf Schwarzer and Matthias Jerusalem) have identified the key aspects of self-belief that we need to be aware of, including the following:

- Feeling positive about your coping skills generally;
- Being able to get what you need from people;
- Being able to solve problems, if you put enough effort in;
- Having the confidence to cope with unexpected events;
- Feeling that you have the resourcefulness to cope with what life throws at you.

Give yourself a rating from 1–10 (1 is low, 10 high) for the five points above. A score below 25 indicates there is scope for you to improve the level of belief in your ability to cope. It is important to work at your coping skills, particularly if you are going through a challenging phase in your life.

63
Track your time

Try tracking if you're often late or miss appointments. Over the course of one day time as many of your daily activities as possible. Tracking your time may quickly reveal some startling truths.

After completing this exercise one of my coaching clients realised that what she thought was only one hour checking her email each day actually amounted to three. She was able to reduce this time significantly and as a consequence got more done.

Hire in help

Ever had the feeling that your to-do list is never ending? The volume of routine tasks on your to-do list may seem harmless but these tasks steal time from the important things. If you could afford it, what activities would you pay someone else to do? Is there a way to start with the least inexpensive activity and hire someone straight away? Can any of your tasks be delegated? Or is there a need to make a decision to stop doing the activity altogether?

Mobilise the time you have

This is particularly important when you have a limited amount of time to complete an action. Have you had plenty of time to meet a deadline and instead found yourself distracted and wasting time? Or maybe you're up against a tight deadline to get a task completed that would on a normal day take double or triple the amount of time? Suddenly you're on top of it. You pull out all the stops and in the time you have the job gets done. You've just experienced what time management gurus refer to as Parkinson's Law. Parkinson's Law can be effectively used in both scenarios by setting aside a certain amount of time that you stick to while you concentrate your focus and get the task completed in the allocated slot of time.

Strategic deceit

This is very useful when it's a challenge to schedule in me-time. Fabricating self-imposed meetings and appointments in your diary is another way of saving time. Writer Heather Sellers calls this 'strategic deceit'. It's not the same as lying but a method used to create time that you wouldn't normally allow yourself to have. What harm would it really do to schedule in the end of a meeting an hour later so you can take an uninterrupted lunch break before rushing back to the office? You're more likely to give yourself permission to time for yourself when you've scheduled it in your diary in the same way you schedule in appointments for clients and other people.

Intelligent neglect

A simple time analysis may reveal the fact that you're spending far too much time on your computer or your mobile phone. Spending less time on the Internet or your mobile phone (even small chunks of time) lowers stress and allows time for reflective thinking and solution solving. Time to think increases productivity and efficiency. In the time management world taking time off from technology is known as the practice of 'intelligent neglect'. It includes regular periods of switching your mobile to voicemail, going through your inbox and unsubscribing from mailing lists, and checking emails only once or twice a day.

64
Revamp your to-do list

To-do lists are essential for most of us but they can be a huge drain on energy.

The list that never seems to get any shorter is not so much an aide-memoire as a horrible reminder that we're running fast but getting nowhere. And what could be more dispiriting than that?

The other side, of course, is that to-do lists are incredibly useful tools for motivating us and making us more productive. Having a clear plan for the day ahead focuses the mind and puts you in control like nothing else. Whether you're a CEO, freelance, stay-at-home parent or student, the well run to-do list will give you a sense of full-capacity living.

But for it to work, you have to have a definite system. Try this one. It is based on the advice given to 1930s magnate Charles Schwabb by a young man he challenged to double his productivity. The young man told him to write down the six most crucial tasks for each day in order of importance and work down the list. Then teach his staff to do the same. After a few weeks, the story goes that Schwabb sent a cheque for £25,000 to the young man, which was a huge sum then.

This idea works on the principle that we put off important stuff (or we work to others' agenda so we don't get round to what's important for us) and keep ourselves busy with lesser tasks to distract ourselves. But if we don't do the one important thing, no matter what we achieve, we'll feel dissatisfied at the end of the day. Instead of an abstract list of things to do that you attack randomly, switch the angle from what you must do to when you are going to do it.

How to revamp your to-do list

In your diary or a separate notebook, draw a line down the left-hand side of the page to form a column and mark in the working hours of the day. This can be precise (9.30 to 10.30, 10.30 to 11.30) or loose (morning, afternoon). Now you're set to go.

- At the end of your working day, brew a cuppa, sit for a second, take a deep breath and gather your thoughts. Pat yourself on the back for what you have achieved today. Now. Swing your mind forward into tomorrow.

- Ask yourself what regular scheduled tasks or meetings you have for tomorrow. Block them off on your diary page.

- Remember to add in travelling time, lunch and relaxation.

- What is your major task? What must you do tomorrow? That gets priority and should be done first thing if possible. Set aside a realistic block of time (err on the side of caution). Be precise.

- Put in specific times for phone calls/emails. It is more time effective to do these in two or three blocks rather than breaking concentration and doing it ad hoc during the day.

- What's your next most important task? Is there room in your day? If you have time left, you can schedule in other tasks, but be realistic.

- For each week have a short list of brief one-off tasks (phone calls, paying bills, birthday cards) and if you have a few down minutes, slot them in.

Simple but effective

Switch off your mobile for as long as you can comfortably get away with, but aim for at least an hour in the morning and an hour in the afternoon. These should be your high productivity times when you aim to really motor through your tasks. The act of switching off your mobile sends an unconscious message to your brain that this is time when your interests are the priority, and it helps to focus your mind on the task at hand.

65
Crisis management

Facing the week from hell? Here's how to survive it. This is the toolbox for navigating through those really stressful, busy times.

Don't catastrophise

Dorothy Parker, on hearing a telephone ring, apparently drawled 'What fresh hell is this?' We've all been there. On really busy days with multiple deadlines, I've got to the stage where I'm scared to answer the phone in case it's someone demanding something else of me. Then I made a conscious decision to stop being such a victim. My attitude became 'Why fear the worse until it happens?' Every time a negative thought crosses your brain, cancel it out with a positive one. This takes practice. An easy way to do it is to develop a mantra to suit whatever crisis you're in today and that you say to yourself mindlessly every time your mind goes into tailspin. Right now, I have to pick the kids up from school in half an hour. I have four weeks to my deadline for this book and I have done approximately half the number of words I promised myself I'd write today. My mantra is 'I am serenely gliding towards my deadline and everything will get done' and every time panic hits, I chant this to myself and feel much better.

Master the only question that matters

The 'best use' question was taught to me by my first boss and it is invaluable in negotiating your way through any day with dozens of calls on your time. It helps you to prioritise 'on the run', sometimes quite ruthlessly. On the morning of manic days decide what you've got to achieve that day and if anything interrupts, ask yourself, 'Is this the best use of my time, right now?' If the answer's no, take a raincheck and come back to it later. So if a friend calls at work, nine times out of ten, you won't chat then, you'll call her back at a more convenient time – unless, of course, she is very upset about something, then talking to her is the best use of your time. Nothing else is more important. By doing this, I don't let colleagues sidetrack me with complaints about their lack of stationery, unless of course it's the best use of my time. (No, you're right, so far stationery has never been the best use of my time, but you get the idea.)

Always underpromise

A lot of stress is of our own making. Thomas Leonard, who founded Coach University, the first professional training centre for life coaches says, 'One of the biggest mistakes is to tell people what they want to hear, give them what they think they want, without thinking if it's feasible for you. You overpromise results you can't deliver without a lot of stress. And of course, if you don't deliver, not only are you stressed, they are, too.' Leonard's advice is to underpromise rather than overpromise. That way your friends are delighted when you turn up at the party you said you couldn't make and your boss thinks you're wonderful when you get the report finished a day early rather than a week late. Make it your rule from now on to be absolutely realistic about how long it's going to take you to get things done. And until you get expert at this, work out the time you reckon it will take you to complete any task and multiply it by 1.5.

Keep a time log of your working week so you finally get a realistic idea of how long it takes you to complete all your usual activities. This means you stop kidding yourself about how quickly you will perform tasks in an imperfect world – where you're interrupted frequently – and you'll reduce your stress levels hugely.

Life events versus daily hassles

It may be that the nature and scale of the situation we are facing is truly threatening, e.g. loss of a loved one, loss of a job, in which case anyone's ability to cope will be severely challenged. These significant life events demand significant efforts to cope with. Psychiatrists, Holmes and Rahe, developed a 'ladder' of life events from the least to the most demanding; the higher up the steps an event is perceived to be, the greater the coping effort required. The impact of these events is cumulative; the more we have to deal with, the more our coping skills are tested. Sometimes we may not realise the magnitude of the challenge we face, until it becomes obvious our attempts to cope are not up to the challenge. Then we need to get help, as the saying goes 'a problem shared is a problem halved', whether that be through social or professional contacts.

Rather than life events, we more often find ourselves dealing with a series of minor issues, which gradually gang up on us and grind us down over a period of time. We tend to forget about these daily hassles, but they too are cumulative and the more we have to deal with, the more our coping skills are tested. Life can keep piling on life events, daily personal and work hassles, so it is not surprising that occasionally our coping skills are overwhelmed – the balance tips and we feel we are no longer coping. Time to get some assistance and engage our coping skills before our sense of well-being is undermined and damaged!

Dealing with bullying

At a psychological level, bullying is an attempt by the bully to get their own way, to put down the competition or in extreme cases they may get satisfaction from making someone else suffer. Their motivation is usually selfish and they do not care about the needs of the other party – in this regard, they are being highly aggressive, i.e. violating another's needs for the benefit of their own. Some bullies are careful about who they bully and how they do it, being careful not to show their hand in public. Others take delight in throwing their weight around in public.

The first step in dealing with a bully is to look at yourself and your own behaviour – bullies often pick people who are more submissive and vulnerable. You need to prepare yourself mentally for asserting your needs and rights in a situation: you have the right to be listened to and to have your views taken account of. Picture yourself as a strong person who has the right to be heard. What words are you going to use? For example, 'I would like to express my concern about the impact of change of team leader … '. What tone of voice and body language are you going to use – will you sit or stand up, will you use your hands to emphasise your point? If necessary repeat yourself (broken record technique). Sometimes highlighting the impact of their behaviour on you can help them realise what they are doing. Recognise they have a right to be heard too and try to take account of their views – then it makes it easier for them to do the same. Essentially you are demonstrating 'appropriate assertiveness' – getting your own needs, rights and wants addressed, while not violating the needs, rights and wants of the other party. You have the right to expect the same from them!

What organisations can do

Most reputable organisations now have policies and procedures for dealing with harassment and bullying, indeed many of them have run 'awareness sessions' for their employees, so everyone knows what it is and understands the associated policies. Often there is a 'zero-tolerance' policy, which means that harassment and bullying are not tolerated in any way and incidents are taken very seriously. If someone is feeling that they are being harassed or bullied, then they have the right to put in a complaint. There are usually two levels of complaint – informal, where the issue is dealt with without resort to a formal investigation through supervised meetings and mediation, and formal, where an official complaint is investigated thoroughly.

66
Leave the office on time

Reduce interruptions. Reclaim your evenings. Take control. Don't let your working day be hijacked by others. The secret is to have your goals clear in your mind.

Think weekly, then daily

Don't be a slave to the daily to-do list. See the big picture. On Monday morning lose the sinking 'I've got so much to do' sensation. Instead, think 'What are my goals for this week?' Decide what you want to have done by Friday and then break each goal into smaller tasks that have to be undertaken to achieve all you want by Friday. Slot these tasks in throughout your week. This helps you prioritise so that the tricky and difficult things, or tasks that depend on other people's input, don't sink to the back of your consciousness. It also means you are giving attention to all that you have to do and not spending too much time on one task at the beginning of the week.

Concentrate on three or four items on your to-do list at once. You won't be overwhelmed.

Work with your energy cycles

Some of us operate better in the morning, some in the late afternoon. If your job demands creativity, block out your most creative periods so that you can concentrate on your projects.

Don't allow them to be impinged upon by meetings and phone calls that could be done any time.

Make the phone call you're dreading

Right now. That call that saps your energy all day. Just do it.

Have meetings in the morning

People are buzzing. They want to whizz through stuff and get on with their day. Morning meetings go much faster than those scheduled in the afternoon.

Check emails three times a day

First thing in the morning, just after lunch and just before you leave are ideal times. Keeping to this discipline means that you don't use email as a distraction.

Limit phone calls

Talk to other people when it suits you, not them. In my working life I receive around twenty phone calls a day. Answer machines don't help me personally – the call-back list is another chore. This is how I turned it around. The most time-effective way of using the phone is to limit your calls as you do your emails – to three times a day. Make a list of calls you have to make that day. Call first thing. If someone isn't there, leave a message and unless you have to talk to them urgently, ask them to call you back at your next 'phone period'. Just before lunch is good. That means neither of you will linger over the call. Your other 'phone time' should be around 4.30 p.m. for the same reason. Of course, you can't limit phone calls completely to these times but most of us have some control over incoming calls. I don't have a secretary any more to screen calls, but I very politely say, 'Sorry, I'm in the middle of something.' I tell the caller when I'll be free and most people offer to call me back then, saving me the hassle of calling them. No one minds that if their call isn't urgent. The point of all this is to keep phone calls shorter by putting them in a context of a busy working day. Social chat is important and nice but most of us spend too much time on it. Time restrictions stop us rambling on. And this goes for personal calls too. Check your watch as soon as a friend calls. Give yourself five minutes maximum. Or better still save personal calls as a treat for a hardworking morning.

Create a 'virtual you' if you're getting stressed out in the office by the demands of others. When you're an administrative lynchpin, set up a shared file where people can go to find the information or resources they'd usually get from you.

67
Love your money

And it will love you right back. And that can only have a positive effect on your well-being.

Quickly, without thinking too much about it, write down three phrases that come into your head when you think about your finances. (Hint. Unless your three words are 'abundant, balanced, life-enhancing', then you need this idea.) This idea is about respect. If you're disrespectful of your money, I'm prepared to bet that money is a stressor in your life. If you don't take care of your money, the chances are that, just like a neglected teenager, it's never going to amount to much. Worse, the relationship will probably deteriorate further. One day your money is going to do the equivalent of coming home pregnant with a crack cocaine habit.

Here's a quick test

Get out your wallet or purse. Check out how it looks. Is it neat with bills folded, receipts tucked away or is it, frankly, a mess?

Here's a quicker one

How much money have you got in your wallet right now? If you're out by more than the price of a coffee, you need this idea badly. Your money is your friend. You should love it like a member of the family. You wouldn't go to the shops and forget to bring home one of the kids. Well, why the hell would you misplace your money?

Look for your latte factor

Make a list of everything you spend in a day. Keep a notebook with you and write down how often you take money out of the 'hole in the wall' and what you spend it on. Every online transaction. Every card you swipe. Every time you spend a penny. Literally. Keep it up for a week, preferably for a month. Now multiply (by 52 or 12). That's what it costs to run your life. Go through and highlight the big essentials – the mortgage, the essential bills. Now get out a calculator and work out what you spend on lunches, clothes, magazines, newspapers.

> Go treasure hunting. Look for money down the side of sofas, in pockets, in foreign currency. How much money have you got stuffed in books. Or unrealised in gift tokens. How much of your money are you ignoring?

You're looking for what has been called 'the latte factor', those items that are completely expendable and add very little to your life but cost a fortune. It will frighten the bejasus out of you. I had a client whose latte factor was £472. I needed that money a whole lot more than Starbuck's. You also realise how much it costs to run your life. The very first day I practised this exercise I spent £197.45. And all I came home with was a pound of cherries. Shocking. We're not going to talk about debt here but if you've got personal debt, do this for a month and you are going to work out exactly why.

Writing down what you spend is a fantastically useful exercise whether you're overspending or not. It sure as hell won't de-stress you in the short term but it will in the long term. It allows you to see almost instantly who or what you're spending your money on and then decide if you're happy with that. It allows you to take control, and every way you can find to foster the illusion of control is helpful if you want to be less stressed. Spiritual teachers tell us that money is neither bad nor good, it's simply a way we register our presence in the world. If you fritter away money as a distraction, you'll never focus long enough to work out what's really important to you. If you spend what you don't have, your spirit as well as your bank balance is going to be overstretched. Your bank balance isn't important. Your spirit is. Respect it, protect it – and you're going to make someone very happy, and that someone isn't your bank manager.

Five ways to get financially organised

Why not keep a spending diary for a month? Write down every penny you spend– everything – from that newspaper, those new shoes, daily cappuccinos, to the bills, mortgage, childcare, meals out. That way you know exactly how much you're spending – and what you can really afford.

Reduce your financial clutter. Buy several files and label them – bills, invoices, pay slips, and receipts (separated into 'clothes,' 'household stuff', 'car' and so on). It's a really effective way to help you keep track of your spending and useful in case you need to change things/take purchases back.

Keep all your receipts and post in one place. Go through these papers every week or so, and file them regularly. Sit down and pay all bills in one go, write 'paid' on each, file them. Assess which bills would be easier to keep track of, plus cheaper, if you paid them by direct debit.

Check your bank statement once or twice a month to keep track of funds. Switching to an online account means you can check it every day and may help get rid of some of that annoying paperwork.

Invest in a shredder for old bank statements/credit card bills so you can bin excess paperwork without worrying who may find your personal details. Recycle the old paper waste. Or start banking and paying bills, etc. online – much easier, less clutter.

68
Soaring self-esteem

We formulate who we are through a lifetime of experience. As children, our self-confidence is either nurtured or destroyed depending on how we interpret events.

I have a friend whose view of men was coloured by her experiences as a five-year-old child.

When on holiday with her parents at the seaside, she formed a play friendship with an older boy who was a skilled sandcastle builder. At the end of the day, having been a very willing assistant to the boy's efforts, my friend thought she deserved at least a kiss. Unsurprisingly the boy wasn't into kissing girls and told her this in no uncertain terms! The sense of rejection she felt has haunted my friend throughout her life. The interpretation she put on this tiny event was that men would reject her.

Unless you have very forward-thinking and sensitive parents who are ready to reinterpret these messages, hundreds of assumptions are formed before we reach adulthood. A teacher could have told you that you'll never amount to anything in your life, or your first boyfriend could have told you that you're fat. The trick is to know that everyone is filtering the 'truth'. In other words, everyone is wearing different, funny-coloured pairs of spectacles and seeing their own version of the truth.

Full house

Getting your own house in order first is the key to self-esteem. Knowing the boundaries of what you will and won't accept is vital. In this way, those around you aren't defining who you are the whole time. If you went by their reflections, you would never know who you're trying to be. You can't please everyone all of the time. The only thing you can do is do the best for yourself and know where your limits are.

Will-o'-the-wisp

Self-confidence is a will-o'-the-wisp that can disappear as fast as you've captured it. The trick is to build on your esteem foundations so that you can refer to your successes and know that you have a core of confidence that will never be knocked. Start building up your own library of successes in your life, from when you won the Tennis Improvement Cup to getting into university. If you can put these mementos into a scrapbook, great. Collect photos and certificates of your glorious moments so that you then have a permanent record of wins that you can go back and refer to, no matter how bad things get in the future.

If your job is eating away at your self-esteem you could change jobs, but your self-esteem might be too low to look at this option just yet. You need to start by changing your attitude. If there's a particular person getting you down then change your attitude towards them. Instead of hating them, make an effort to be extra helpful and extra nice. Go the extra mile! Disarm them with your charm! Pretend that you're confident, even if you're not. Everyone is doing this and people who come across as confident are often the ones who feel they don't have a clue what they're doing and are terrified of being found out!

If your partner is denting your confidence by always putting you down look at your boundaries. It's very important to know where you begin and your partner ends. Perfect partnerships are about being a team and each team member has something unique to contribute. If everybody did the same thing in the same way, we wouldn't get very far. I'd suggest becoming gently assertive, which isn't the same as being aggressive. Being assertive is knowing what your needs are and gently getting them. The biggest word in an assertive person's vocabulary is 'No.'

Finally, if you feel that this confidence thing is not something you can gain on your own, you could work with a life coach. But fundamentally, nobody can *give* you confidence. You have to believe in yourself, your values and where you stand and don't be swayed by anyone telling you that you can't be an extraordinary human being. As the Buddha said, 'Peace comes from within. Do not seek it without.'

Get some perspective and start looking up rather than down! I mean this literally. Stop spending so much of your time thinking about the past and future and looking down at your boots. Spend a day looking up instead and see how much more positive you feel about life. Look at your body and how you're holding yourself. Stop slouching otherwise you'll feel like a slouch. Stand up tall, put your shoulders back and smile. Acting as if you were confident will work quickly and effectively to elevate your self-esteem.

69
Achieve the life–work balance in ten minutes

You'll usually see it referred to as work–life balance but it should be life–work. And that's what achieving it entails – a life-work. Unless of course, you've read this idea.

One of the most pernicious things about stress is the way we don't notice how it switches our attention away from what we value and love in life until it's too late. So here are some clues to work out if stress is stomping all over your life–work balance…

- Do you feel like your day is spent dealing with difficult people and difficult tasks?

- Do you feel that those you love don't have a clue what's going on with you and you don't have a clue what's going on with them?

- Do you regularly make time for activities that nourish your soul?

- Do you feel you could walk out the door of your house and no one would notice you were gone until the mortgage had to be paid?

Yes, you guessed it? Number 3 was the trick question. Answer yes to that one and you're probably all right. Answer yes to the rest and you could be in trouble.

In a nutshell: make sure you're putting time and effort into the people and activities that make your heart sing and it really is very difficult to buckle under the effect of stress.

But perhaps too much emphasis is put on the stress caused by the 'work' part of the equation and not enough placed on the stress caused by the 'life' bit. Everyone assumes that all we need is less work, more life and all would be harmonious balance. Hmmm.

Where it has gone all wrong for so many, women especially, is that they've cleared enough time for the 'life' part of the equation but not taken into account that it isn't necessarily restful or enjoyable. This is no idle observation. Research shows that men's stress hormones tend to fall when they get home whereas women's stay high after the working day, presumably because they get home to confront a dozen chores and hungry kids. Your children may be the reason you get out of bed in the morning, but you need to accept that spending time with them is not necessarily any less stressful than work – in fact, it often makes work seem like a walk in the park. More time with your kids is not necessarily the answer.

More time with yourself, very probably, is.

That old saw is true – if you don't look after yourself, you can't look after anyone else. And all it takes is just ten minutes a day.

And ten minutes of selfishness every day is enough to make a profound difference in your ability to achieve a life balance that works. Try it.

Designate Saturday 'family' day and Sunday afternoon 'selfish' time. We can usually find an hour or so on Sunday afternoon to spend on ourselves – just don't let it get filled with chores or your partner's agenda.

Have a very clear list in your head of what is important to you. Instead of abstract virtues (integrity, passion), work out your different roles and their importance in your life. My roles at the moment are: wife, mother, employee, author, student, counsellor, daughter, sister, friend ... You get the idea, note down yours. Stop at ten. Then prioritise them. You won't always stick to this order but it will give you a working template that you can use when you are running around like a headless chicken and don't know where to turn.

When we're living a life out of balance, life is tougher. When we're clear about what's important and focusing on it, life flows more smoothly.

70

Keeping your relationship minty-fresh

Read, digest and ponder. Then get your diary, a big red pen and start prioritising your relationship.

This chapter contains the three golden rules of a healthy relationship. Couples that spend time together, and anticipate and plan for those times, find it hard to lose interest in one another.

Rule 1: daily...

How is your partner feeling right now? What's happening at work? How are their relationships with friends, colleagues, siblings, parents? Carve out fifteen minutes of every day to talk. If you find yourselves getting into a rut of busy-ness, when you pass like ships in the night for several days in a row without touching base, either go to bed before your usual time or get up earlier and have a coffee together so you can touch base.

Kiss each other every morning before you get out of bed. Take the time for a swift cuddle. Breathe deeply. Hold tight. Do the same at night. Never take your physical intimacy for granted. In this Vale of Tears we call life, you found each other. Pretty amazing. Worth acknowledging that with at least a daily hug, methinks.

Rule 2: weekly...

Go out with each other once a week where humanly possible. Once a fortnight is the bare minimum. According to the experts, this is the most important thing you can do. Couples who keep dating, keep mating. Spending too long sloping around the same house does something to a couple's sexual interest in each other and what it does generally isn't good. So get out, preferably after making some small effort to tart yourself up so you're visually pleasing to your partner. Let them see why they bothered with you in the first place. (No, I never said this chapter was rocket science. I just said that it worked.)

Look for easy ways to cheer your partner up. Pick up a tub of her favourite ice-cream on the way home from work. Run him a bath and bring him a beer. Sappy gestures work – they build up a huge bank of goodwill that couples can draw on when life gets stressful.

You don't have to go out for long – an hour or two is fine. Even parents of newborns can find a way if sufficiently motivated.

- No money? Make it a challenge to have a good night out on a tenner or less. If all else fails, go for a walk and treat yourself to half a pint of lager at your local. Oh OK, share half a pint if money's really tight.

- No childcare? Make it your mission to seek out other couples with kids who live locally – ideally, in the next street – and look like they enjoy going out (single parents and confirmed stay-at-homes are no good for this). The deal is that one half of their couple comes to your house and sits with your kids once a week. The next week one of you returns the favour. It means that for one night's babysitting you get two nights out and an evening home alone. Not bad.

- No conversation? You'd better fix this one before you do anything else.

Rule 3: monthly…

Go for a mini-adventure – shared memories cement your relationship. Make your adventure as mad or staid as you like, but at the least make sure it's something that you haven't done since the beginning of your relationship. It really doesn't matter what it is, as long as it's not your usual 'date'. Here's a year's worth:

- hill walking between two cosy pubs;
- hiring some cycles;
- al fresco dining, with champagne and strawberries;
- horse riding;
- paragliding;
- spending a weekend in a city you've never visited before;
- punting along a river or taking out a rowing boat in your local park;
- watching a matinée at the cinema;
- spending a day at a health spa;
- visiting an art gallery;
- going to the theatre;
- attending a self-help seminar.

Take turns to suggest the adventure, and go along with your partner's choice even if you don't fancy it. Even the disasters will give you shared memories to laugh about afterwards.

What's the point? You see your partner coping with new environments and new skills and that keeps you interested in them. And them in you. Simple.

If you're shaking your head and tutting 'how banal', I'd get that smug look off your face, pronto. Research shows quite clearly that one of the defining differences between strong couples and 'drifting' couples is the amount of effort and time they spend on their shared pursuits. All of us have heard the advice, 'Spend more time with each other being as interesting as possible.' But how many couples do you know who actually do it? I'm prepared to bet that those who do seem happiest.

71

Avoid the brain drain

Are you feeling mentally sluggish? Having difficulty concentrating? Got an important exam or interview coming up, but feel like your brain has all the sharpness of a wet sponge?

We can help. In just two weeks.

Brain ageing starts at a very young age, far younger than most of us imagine. How young? Your twenties, basically. No sooner has your brain stopped growing (late teens, early twenties) than it starts deteriorating. Ironic? No kidding. But given there's not much mileage in railing against evolution, what can we do about it?

A lot is the answer. Genetics is only about one-third of what predicts brain ageing, say the boffins at UCLA's Anti-Ageing Institute. The other two-thirds have to do with our environment and lifestyle choices.

Retrain your brain

If you're mentally sluggish and have trouble remembering not just where you left the car keys, but where you left the car, try this programme based on the latest research into brain drain. You can hope to see more mental sharpness within a few weeks.

Every morning

Chuck a handful of blueberries, prunes or raisins onto your

porridge. These and other fruits and vegetables which have a deep-blue colour are particularly high on the 'ORAC scale'. The higher it is on the ORAC scale, the more brain-boosting anti-ageing antioxidants a food has.

Every day

Eat three meals and two snacks. Your brain needs a steady flow of glucose. Aim for at least one food supplying omega-3 oils – that's avocados, walnuts and of course, fish. Or pop a supplement – either fish oil or flax seed oil if you're a vegetarian. Limit saturated fatty foods – red meat and dairy.

Every couple of hours

De-stress. Cortisol is released when we're stressed and, according to experts constant stress shrinks a key memory centre in the brain. Every hour or so, stand up, take a deep breath and raise your arms above your head. Exhale and drop your arms. Repeat three times. This de-stresses your brain and your body as well as sending oxygen to your brain.

Every two or three days

Go for a walk Walking every two or three days for ten minutes, building up to forty-five minutes, was found to result in an improvement in mental agility. Stretching and toning exercises did not have this effect.

Health journalists have been twittering on for years about how doing puzzles like crosswords keeps the mind active into old age. It appears that we're wrong. Research does show that the brain can be retrained right into your eighties to learn new languages and skills – or indeed, how to do crosswords – but University of Virginia research shows that while mental challenges will keep you competent at doing those particular mental challenges, they will not necessarily stop Alzheimer's.

However, you can become sharper at mental challenges by practising. For instance, if you want to become better at sitting multiple-choice exams, guess what? Repeatedly practising multiple-choice questions will make you faster and better at them.

Improve your concentration

Stick on some Mozart. Research from the University of California shows that people who listened to Sonata for Two Pianos in D Major while preparing for an IQ test scored higher than those who studied in silence. Mozart is the gold standard, but any rhythmic music will help as long as it doesn't have lyrics that disrupt concentration.

Set your brain a goal. Recall what the first three people you see were wearing. If you're told a phone number, work out a memory aide so you can dial it later. Invent another to help you remember the name of anyone you're introduced to (for example, if their name is Baker, imagine a loaf of bread on their head).

Give your brain a rest

Research at the prestigious Tufts University in the States discovered that people who sit quietly for ten minutes a day, observing their heart rate on a monitor and concentrating on lowering it, had reduced anxiety and increased feelings of well-being and energy. Here are four 'brain holidays'. Build these into your day as often as you remember. Aim for two minutes, building up to ten:

- Try sitting quietly taking your pulse and concentrating on slowing it down (it doesn't matter if you don't; it's the concentration that counts).

- Take a look out of the window. Observe what you see but don't react to it. When you do react (for example, you can't help getting upset when you see someone drop litter outside your gate), notice your reaction and then let it float away like a cloud.

- The easiest meditation of all. Breathe. Just as normal, don't change a thing. Observe your breath. Notice how the air is cooler as it enters your nostrils and that it is warmer when you exhale. Feel the air reaching your lungs. Notice how your belly expands as you inhale, flattens as you exhale. When your mind wanders, notice it and bring it back to the breath.

- Light a candle, watch the flame. Concentrate on the flame and bring your mind back to it when it wanders off.

72
A one-minute answer to mid-afternoon slump

Practically every medical system in the world (with the exception of our own) believes that energy flows around the body in channels. Lack of energy is attributed to a block somewhere in this energy flow. Release the block and you get increased energy. You can do this by applying needles, fingers or elbows to specific acupuncture points around the body.

True? Or unmitigated waffle? Here we're dealing with acupressure and there isn't scientific evidence that would pass muster with the *British Medical Journal* when it comes to acupressure and energy. However, there is evidence that acupressure works for helping with post-operative nausea and lower back pain – so working on the principle that if it works for one thing it may work for another, it's worth a try. I have derived benefit from the following facial massage which is specifically for tiredness and mental exhaustion. It was taught to me by a TCM (traditional Chinese medicine) doctor about twenty years ago. There may be a placebo effect going on here, but hey, who cares? Whatever gets you through the night or, in this case, through the afternoon. This is brilliant for mid-afternoon slump. I've since taught it to friends – specifically those who spend a lot of time at their desk– and many use it.

Shiatsu facial massage for instant energy

Lean your elbows on a table and let your face drop into your hands, with your palms cupped over your eyes. Look into the darkness formed by your hands. Stay there for as long as you feel comfortable or until your colleagues start to get worried.

Place your thumbs on the inner end of each eyebrow and use your index fingers to work out along the upper edge of the eyebrow, applying pressure at regular intervals. When your index fingers reach the outer edge of your eyebrow, release all pressure.

Return index finger to the inner end of each brow and work thumbs along to the lower end of the brows in similar fashion. Release as before.

Place thumbs under ear lobes and apply pressure. At the same time, use the index fingers to apply pressure on points on a line from the bridge of the nose under your eyes, along the ridge formed by your eye sockets.

Touch fingertips to fingertips along an imaginary line running up the middle of your forehead from your nose to your hairline (no pressure is necessary). Use thumbs to apply pressure to points fanning out from the outer edge of the eyebrows to hairline. Repeat four times. (Feel for tender points and massage them. I find pressing on my temples when I'm stressed decreases tension in my jaw where, like a lot of people, I hold a lot of tension.)

Use thumbs to apply gentle pressure in the eye sockets under the inner end of the eyebrow where you feel a notch at the ridge of the eye socket. (This is a very delicate spot. I was told by a doctor once that it is the closest major nerve to the surface of the body: I don't know if that's true, but go gently. You can really hurt yourself by pressing this point too hard.)

Use one index finger to work up that imaginary line in your mid-forehead from the nose to your hairline.

Now drop your head forward and, lifting your arms, work

thumbs from your spine outwards along the ridge of your skull, from the spine out to the point just under your earlobes. Do this four times.

OK, it's a bit of a faff to get the hang of the different points, but once you've practised a couple of times with the instructions, you'll have the hang of it. And it will be a good friend to your energy levels for the rest of your life.

If mid-afternoon tiredness gets you down, combine the massage with this energising meditation – or do this instead of it. Empty your brain as far as possible, sit quietly, get an orange and concentrate on peeling it. Look at it first – orange is an energising colour. Smell it – citrus scents such as orange, bergamot and lemon are revitalising. Eat it – vitamin C and fructose make a wicked combination for energy. After your orange, drink a large glass of water. You should feel better in ten minutes.

73
Energise your work life

Let's face it – the daily grind of work or life's routines does sap our morale at times. That comfortable groove can turn into a rut that we cannot escape from. The sparkle can go out of our lives, if you do not work at it. We need to listen to our needs, take a bit of sagely advice from well-being experts and then have the discipline to put that advice into practice.

Focus on what you do well and start your day with what you feel you are really good at. It may sound indulgent, but a reputable researcher into depression, Martin Seligman has consistently shown that people who focus on their 'signature strengths' are generally significantly more satisfied and less depressed. So all you managers out there – help your team to focus on what they are good at and you will reap the rewards of having satisfied, productive colleagues. A great start, but you can do more!

More healthy advice from Seligman – review what has gone well at the end of a day or the start of the new day. It is a variation on the theme of 'counting your blessing', but focused on what you contributed positively to people and relationships, what you achieved and what meant something to you.

All this advice is geared towards building your positive emotions in the workplace and thereby helping to create a 'virtuous, energising cycle'. There are plenty of 'energy vampires' out there, so take more control of energising yourself and tap into what makes you feel enthused and happy.

Five ways to energise your work life

- Ignore the view of the car park. Exposure to a 'natural scene' is an excellent antidote to mental fatigue. Get to the park if you can at lunch or pin up some beautiful pictures of green countryside above your desk.

- Remember the 90:120 rule. Plan your working day in 120-minute blocks. US research shows that somewhere between 90 and 120 minutes we lose focus. After 90 minutes, stop, take a few minutes to walk around, stretch, drink a glass of water or have a cup of tea. When you return to work do another sort of task until the 120-minute mark – email, make calls or switch to another job. After two hours, plan what to do for the next 120-minute block. You'll find that you have more momentum and are more productive.

- Open mail standing next to the waste paper bin and throw out rubbish then and there.

- Keep a notebook with you and write down every potential task as it pops into your brain – this brings home to you that you almost certainly can't do it all. You have to pick and choose.

- Don't screen calls – you only have to call the people back later. But if you have to screen, set aside a slot at the end of the day to make calls. A bad conscience is an energy drain.

74
Let in the light

Most of us have heard of SAD – Seasonal Affective Disorder – but are less aware that there are millions of people affected by the 'sub-syndrome'. They don't have SAD, but they feel exhausted all winter.

Before electricity, our ancestors' life changed completely as they went through the winter. Lack of daylight affected every part of their lives. Now we can work and play round the clock; the lack of light need never impinge on our 'lifestyle'.

But that doesn't mean that lack of daylight doesn't have a profound effect on us.

Normal electric lights can't replace daylight as far as our bodies are concerned, which explains why millions of us suffer symptoms of SAD unwittingly. And lack of energy is one of the biggest symptoms.

Around one in twenty of us suffer from SAD, which can involve severe depression, but what's amazing is that so many of us don't realise it and a far, far larger number are believed by experts to suffer from a milder form without ever knowing it. And lack of energy is the clearest symptom of this 'sub-syndrome'.

- Do you dread the winter months?

- Do you feel lethargic during the months of November to April for no apparent reason?

- Do you tend to put on weight in winter?

- Do you find it near impossible to get out of bed in the morning when it's dark outside?

- Do you find you are more paranoid or self-doubting in winter?

- Do you feel more anxious in winter?

Answer yes to two or more and there's every chance you could be affected by SAD.

The further north you live, the more likely you are to be affected by the lack of light. One study has shown that those in the north-east of Scotland have a higher level of SAD symptoms than average, and it is likely that depression in winter gets gradually more likely the farther north you live, as the light available diminishes.

What can you do?

Stage 1

Get outside for half an hour a day during the winter. Make it a habit of going for a walk at lunchtime, but since sunlight is so precious in the UK during winter, if at all possible, think about dropping everything, making your excuses and getting outside as soon as the sun comes out, whatever time of the day.

Stage 2

If you still feel blue, St John's Wort has been proven to help with the symptoms of SAD. It is not suitable for those on some other medications including the Pill and some heart drugs. It is also helpful in combating the comfort eating that goes along with mild depression.

Stage 3

Investing in a light box, which supplies doses of strong white light as you work, or sit in your home, could well be the answer. A study published in the *American Journal of Psychiatry* found that light therapy was more effective than Prozac in treating SAD: 95 per cent of its users reported that it improved their condition. In general, 85 per cent appear to benefit from light boxes and see an improvement within three to four days of treatment of around two hours a day. Specialised light boxes can be found on the internet, but lights are now readily available on your high street, at chemists and health shops. For milder cases there are 'alarm clocks' that wake you gently and gradually in the morning with light rather than ringing.

Stage 4

If depression is a problem, the group of antidepressants that work best are the SSRIs (Selective Serotonin Reuptake Inhibitors). Older kinds such as the tricyclics tend to make you feel more lethargic and tired, so they aren't the best option if you are already tired.

Drink it in

Have your morning cuppa outside if at all possible, or next to a bright window. Research on sheep in the Western Isles has led scientists to believe that SAD is related to levels of melatonin, the hormone that induces sleep. We need daylight to 'switch off' melatonin after a night's sleep, and getting outside as soon after you wake (as long as it's light, of course) may help.

75
Tired ... or ill?

Yes, you're tired. You're always tired. And now you're beginning to wonder if it could be a sign of something more sinister ...

How can you tell the difference between the sort of tiredness that means you've been overdoing it and the sort of tiredness that means you're ill?

Action plan

1. If persistent tiredness is accompanied by pain or unexplained weight loss, you should see your doctor as soon as possible for a check-up. The two most overlooked causes of unexplained tiredness are reaction to medication (including alternative therapies) – and not realising you're pregnant. Discount both first.

2. Go back to energy basics. The most common causes of exhaustion in youngish adults is lack of good quality sleep, lack of space in your life, and lack of good food. After two weeks of TLC, see your doctor if still tired to explore the following illnesses.

What kind of tired are you?

A gradual-onset tiredness that creeps up on you.

Anything else?

Needing to go to the loo more often, excessive thirst, weight loss, genital itching or thrush.

Could be?

Diabetes. Diabetes is the disease with a 'silent million' sufferers. A million have it; another million are undiagnosed. It's also a disease on the rise; sedentary lifestyles and an overdependence on processed food are contributing factors and more people than ever in their forties are discovering they've got it. If you are over forty, or you have other risk factors such as a family history or being overweight, your doctor should be happy to test you for diabetes if you suspect it's at the root of your tiredness.

What kind of tired?

Lethargic and having difficulty concentrating.

Anything else?

Shortness of breath, dizziness.

Could be?

Anaemia. The tissues of your body need oxygen, which is carried to them by the red blood cells. Red blood cells need iron, so shortage of iron is one cause of anaemia. Menstruating women are most at risk, but anyone can get anaemia, especially if their diet isn't supplying enough iron. Eat more iron-rich food – red meat, fortified cereals and dried fruit – and take a multivitamin with iron in it. The medical line is that you have to have full-blown anaemia to suffer from chronic tiredness, but a study showed that, when iron was given for unexplained tiredness to non-anaemic women, their tiredness diminished. Technically this was the placebo response in action, but the researchers concluded that, since many of these non-anaemic women had low iron (just not enough to be clinical), low-grade iron deficiency could still cause symptoms.

Wash down iron-supplying foods with a glass of orange juice: vitamin C helps iron absorption. (Don't take iron supplements without checking with your doctor first.)

What kind of tired?

Slow, sluggish, everything is in slow motion.

Anything else?

Feeling cold, depression, weight gain, dry, thickened skin.

Could be?

Hypothyroidism. This is a growing problem and the trouble is not in treatment, but in diagnosis. The symptoms start so slowly that often they are misdiagnosed as another disease, for instance, depression or the menopause. If you suspect hypothyroidism, and you're in your forties or fifties, ask your doctor to test your thyroid hormone levels. Replacement hormones can then be prescribed if a deficiency is found. Younger women may have to exclude other diseases before their doctor is willing to test them.

What kind of tired?

You're tired all day despite sleeping at night. Or perhaps you can't sleep at night. On waking, the thought of the day ahead is exhausting.

Anything else?

Lack of joy and motivation, anxiety, sleep problems, loss of libido, lack of interest in your life, eating too much or too little.

Could be?

Depression. Exhaustion is one of the prime symptoms of depression. However, depressed people can help themselves by taking a little gentle exercise every day. Exercise has been proven to improve mood and it will help you sleep at night – good because insomnia makes you even more isolated. Your GP can help with antidepressants and perhaps by offering counselling and other alternatives to drugs. There is a wealth of advice available now that the stigma associated with depression is disappearing.

76
End 'stop and collapse' syndrome

You take holidays. You know how important this is if you want to be stress-free. And then you spend the first week in bed recovering from some dreaded lurgy. You've got leisure sickness – aka 'stop and collapse' syndrome.

The guy who first identified leisure sickness was a sufferer. Professor Ad Vingerhoets of Tilburg University noticed he always got ill on the first days of his holiday. So he did a study of nearly 2,000 men and women aged between 16 and 87. And guess what? He wasn't alone. A small but significant number of his subjects regularly got ill at the weekend or on holidays. (I think his numbers must be an underestimate because most of the people I know are affected.) He discovered that those who got leisure sickness complained mainly of headaches, migraine, fatigue, muscular pains, nausea, colds and flu (especially common when going on holiday).

Those who got it shared certain characteristics: a high workload, perfectionism, eagerness to achieve, an overdeveloped sense of responsibility to their work – all of which makes it difficult to switch off.

One theory is that those who work hard simply get so bored on holiday that they start to notice the symptoms they've been suppressing while at work. It could also be a case of 'mind over matter': we don't allow ourselves to get sick until the work is done. Yet another theory is that when you're working (stressed) the high cortisol (stress hormone) levels affect how your immune system functions. When you relax, the cortisol drops, and with it your defences, and kaboom, you're calling the concierge for a doctor.

So what can you do about it? I'm going to suggest a two-pronged attack.

1. Support your local immune system

As a very bare minimum, eat five fruit and veg a day (you should be aiming for even more than this – many nutritionists reccommend nine – so don't think you should stop at five) and take a good-quality multivitamin and mineral supplement. If you drink too much alcohol or are a smoker, you also need more vitamin C – so supplement that too. I'm also a fan of echinacea, so give this a try as well (but read the instructions carefully: if you take it for too long, it loses its effectiveness).

2. Plan for holidays with military precision

You really need gradually to begin to wind down in the two weeks before you go.

Cue hollow laughter. You think I don't understand, but I do. In August 1998, the day before my holiday, I worked in the office from 6 a.m. until 11 p.m., went home, packed, slept for three hours, went back to the office at 4 a.m., worked until 8.30 and took a cab straight to the airport to get on a plane. That's not smart. That's borderline lunacy. So let's have no more of the workaholic nuttiness.

Here are some ideas (I am assuming everyone in your household has a valid passport. Young children's passports don't run as long as adults. Not sure about this? Go and check right now. This one small action could save you bucketloads of stress down the line.)

Three weeks before you go. Make a packing list. Write down

everything you need to take with you and then allocate each lunchtime this week to completing any errands.

Two weeks before you go. Sort out work. Take a look at all your projects and decide what stage you want to pass them over. Set goals with each project and allocate deadlines for reaching them preferably all to be tied up the day before your last day.

One week before you go. Start packing. Put out your bags or suitcases in a spare room if you've got one and start the washing and ironing nightmare in the weekend before you go. Do a little packing each night. Also start winding up projects and writing up your handover notes to whichever colleague is taking over your responsibilities. You can always amend them on the last day if you get further with a project than you planned to. Amending is a lot better than starting them at 8.30 p.m. on your last day.

If you're prone to weekend sickness, try exercising on a Friday evening. Exercise is a stressor but one your body loves. This acts as a transition between work and time off, and helps you unwind quicker.

77
Don't give up giving up

Quitting for good might seem like climbing Everest. With careful planning, Everest is climbed all the time, and sometimes without oxygen masks. Breaking down stopping into stages can bring the seemingly impossible within your grasp.

Why did you start smoking? To fit in? To look cool? To be grown up? What still applies? What else have you found that smoking does to you, and is it nice? Only you will know the answers to these questions, so why not jot them down? Once you have a list of all the reasons why you want to give up smoking, put the list in your packet and read it through before you light up. Don't deny yourself any cigarettes at this stage.

Preparing to stop

Mess around with your usual smoking routines. If you usually smoke last thing at night, take the dog out for a final walk instead. If you have two smoking breaks at work, try having them both in the morning and introduce a tea break in the afternoon. At this stage, you don't need to focus on smoking any less, just mess around with your habit. Once you've changed your habits, it's easier to break them.

Next you'll be ready to pick a quit date on your calendar and circle it in your favourite colour. Select your preferred way of quitting and buy any aids you might need, like nicotine gum.

Set yourself some goals. It's important that they're specific and attainable. For instance, the goal 'I want to be a non-smoker for good' may be too non-specific and difficult if you've been a heavy smoker all your adult life. 'I want to get through the weekend without smoking' is a more realistic start and means you won't be setting yourself up to fail.

Recruit friends and family, and tell them of your intentions. Be really clear about what you expect from them by way of support. Are you looking for loved ones to be firm with you if your resolve wavers, or will that just draw you into unproductive arguments? Many people find it helps if their families take a positive caring stance without being too judgemental if things don't work out at the first attempt or even fortieth.

Compile a list of useful numbers and keep them by the phone for crisis times ahead. Numbers you might like to have handy are your local quitline, any friends who are also giving up and successful ex-smokers who'll know exactly how you feel and how to get through it.

Stopping

Try to make your quit date as relaxed and stress free as possible. You might like to have a day off and be pampered at a health farm, or you may prefer to throw yourself into work and distract yourself from smoking as much as possible. Whatever you decide, it's vital that you throw away all your cigarettes. No ifs and butts. You've passed the point of no return. It's also time to bin all your lighters and matches. You might want to give the pub a miss for a few weeks, as drink often dilutes the most steadfast resolve.

Beware of substitutes such as e-cigarettes. They may contain fewer chemicals than conventional cigarettes but the flavours do still contain chemicals and the jury is still out regarding the harm they cause, with some early studies suggesting they may cause heart problems or even certain cancers.

Staying stopped

You've done the hard bit, but now you've got to stay strong and stay motivated. Remember why you gave up in the first place; feel proud of what you've achieved so far; change your routine to avoid those smoking triggers; and put the support network that you set up to work.

Relapsing

Relax. These things happen. Many ex-smokers gave up several times before managing to stay stopped for good. The most important thing you can do is recognise it for what it is – a temporary lapse – and start thinking about stopping again. Use your past attempts to help future efforts. What worked last time? How did you successfully cope with cravings? What are the social pressures that make you reach for a smoke? When you gave up last time, how did you cope with your smoking triggers without smoking?

When you relapse, it's tempting to think of it as an all-or-nothing failure. 'What the heck, I've had one, I may as well smoke the whole packet.' Nothing could be further from the truth. If you smoke one cigarette, that's all you've done, smoked a measly cigarette. Why let it beat you? The fewer cigarettes you smoke and the sooner you think about stopping again the better. After all, practice makes perfect.

78
Wired!

After your first sip of coffee you change from a woolly headed, dozy person to a sharp individual ready to meet the challenges of the day.

Why is it that the very things that help you stay alert are going to ruin your chances of a decent night's sleep? Life's just so unfair…

Caffeine

Your morning coffee works for a reason. Caffeine stimulates the central nervous system (brain and spinal chord), increasing your metabolic rate, blood pressure, heart rate, and breathing levels. It also blocks the effects of adenosine, a natural sedative found in the brain which builds up during the day and triggers the adrenal glands to produce the stimulating hormone adrenaline. It works fast, too. Caffeine, which is found in coffee, tea, cola and chocolate, is absorbed in only 15–30 minutes but its effects can last longer than four hours.

No wonder caffeine makes it more difficult to get to sleep and reduces the quality of sleep. Studies show that having a caffeinated drink at night makes you wake up more often – it's particularly thought to reduce deep sleep and REM sleep.

Cutting down:

- Limit yourself to two cups of coffee or three or four of tea, but don't have them too late in the day.

- If you're relying on coffee to give you energy, go for snacks such as a banana, dried fruit or cereal bar, which will do the trick just as well.

- Replace one of your daily teas or coffees with an alternative. Choose from herbal tea, milkshake, fruit juice, smoothie or even decaffeinated tea or coffee.

Alcohol

If you've had a few drinks, you're not likely to have much trouble getting to sleep – probably on the stairs on the way up to bed. But you'll probably wake up again as alcohol has just as disruptive an effect on sleep as caffeine. Although it's a sedative, it causes the release of adrenaline and blocks tryptophan, which helps the body make the calming brain chemical serotonin – vital for sleep. One unit of alcohol (half a pint of beer, one small glass of wine) takes about one hour to metabolise. So if you drink three glasses of wine at 10 p.m., expect your sleep to be disrupted from around 1 a.m. Again some people metabolise it faster than others.

Cutting down

- Have at least two drink-free days a week.

- Don't drink more than two units of alcohol per day if you're a women, three units if you're a man.

- Alternate an alcoholic drink with a non-alcoholic one such as non-alcoholic beer, water or a soft drink.

- Sip your drink slowly so it lasts longer.

- Try to eat before you go drinking since it will help reduce the amount of alcohol absorbed by your body.

Nicotine

The increased risk of cancer and heart disease not a good enough reason to make you give up smoking? Well, this one might.

The average smoker takes twice as long to fall asleep as a non-smoker and sleeps 30 minutes less. You may feel relaxed after having a cigarette, but it's probably because you've satisfied the craving rather than anything in nicotine. In fact, like caffeine it's a powerful stimulant and triggers the release of adrenaline. Like alcohol, once metabolised, nicotine can wake you up. Nicotine can cause difficulty falling asleep, problems waking in the morning, and may also cause nightmares.

Cutting down

There's no cutting down, you've got to bite the bullet and quit.

- If you're a woman, don't pack it in in the second half of your menstrual cycle, though. Researchers have found that you're much more likely to succeed if you do it in the first half because nicotine withdrawal symptoms – depression, anxiety and irritability – are worse in the second half.

- If you can use simply willpower, that's great. Otherwise there's a host of options from nicotine patches and self-help manuals to acupuncture and hypnotherapy. None of these will work unless you really want to give up.

The beginner's guide to napping

- Find somewhere quiet.

- If you're working in an office, switch your phone to voicemail and either sit at your desk or find an empty room. Ideally you'd hang a sign on your door saying 'Do not disturb' and get your secretary to wake you 20 minutes later. But we're not all company directors.

- Loosen your clothing and take off your shoes. Lie down on a sofa, stretch out on the floor or if that's not possible sit comfortably on a chair, placing your head in your folded arms on your desk.

- Close your eyes – ideally, put on an eye mask.

- Try not to think about work or all the things you have to do. Focus on what you love doing in your spare time. If you like golf, you might mentally play a round of golf on your regular course. Maybe drift back to a favourite holiday, or listen to some calming music.

- Just rest at first – if your brain needs a rest as well, you'll soon fall asleep.

- If you do nap, set an alarm clock to wake you up 20 minutes later. Don't sleep for more than 30 minutes – you'll wake up groggier and foggier.

- When you wake up lie still for a minute or two – then stretch and breathe deeply and take a drink of water or a light snack to get your system going again.

- Then, return to work, starting with simple chores such as opening letters or organising the work you have to do. Within just a few minutes you should feel sparky again.

- Download the pzizz app to aid napping and sleeping.

79
Look on the bright side

It's what used to be called PMA – 'positive mental attitude', now more commonly known as 'optimistic thinking'.

There are some people who view the world as full of exciting opportunities or those with their glass 'half full'. There are people who tend to anticipate the worst or those with their glass 'half empty'. Whatever the state of your glass, psychologists have shown that there are significant differences in the way we appraise our lives, ourselves and what happens to us. And what's more intriguing, is that our appraisals have been shown to affect our thinking, our emotions and ultimately our behaviour. Sometimes our negative thinking can actually affect our morale, esteem and mental health.

Taking some lessons from Cognitive Behavioural Therapy (CBT), we need to become aware of our mental dialogue and if we are thinking negatively, we need to try to switch to a more positive appraisal of ourselves and our situation, literally by writing our thoughts down. For example, when hearing bad news about a job promotion:

Self 1   My manager dislikes me, I knew I was not up to it, I will never get a promotion now.

Self 2   It's disappointing that I was not ready this time, but I've learned a lot and will develop myself over the next year.

You can see that the second thought leads to a more positive emotional reaction, disappointment, yes, but focusing on what can be done and a constructive way forward. The ability to manage our own thinking and thereby our feelings is a key life skill and something we all need to work at to keep mentally healthy, particularly in times of austerity and hardship.

80
Working your purpose out

My particular purpose in life is lifting your game. What's yours?

You get out of bed, put the cereal in the toaster and the milk on the toast, and pat the wife and kiss the dog as you leave for work. You have a dark suspicion lurking deep within you. Is this it? Is this all I can expect?

You don't have to be a slave to your job. But knowing what you don't want to do is the easy part of the equation. The tough bit is deciding just what would make you happy. Working with a life coach is a great way to force yourself to face these big questions head on.

Coaching is a relatively new concept that has exploded into quite a movement over the last five years, to the point where in certain circles anyone who is anyone is working with a coach. Coaching shouldn't be confused with mentoring. A mentor is someone who is, for example, a leader in your field who will tell you how to avoid pitfalls and to avoid making the same mistakes as they did. A coach, on the other hand, doesn't 'tell' you to do anything. Coaching works by asking you the right questions so that you can find the answer yourself. As the saying goes, 'Give a man a fish he eats for a day but teach him how to fish and you feed him for life.' There's no point in a coach telling you what to do unless you want to live the coach's life and not your own. Coaching isn't a counselling process either. It assumes that you're healthy in mind and ready to move on from your past and into your future.

You might think that you have lots of friends who could do the same job as a coach but for free, but remember that all of your friends have a vested interest in keeping you just where you are now. They won't usually want you to move on as they like you just the way you are, plus you might show them up for being stuck where they are. Imagine that you tell your best mate that you're considering starting a new life in Spain. 'Oh', he says, 'I heard a story once about someone moving to Spain that would make your hair curl...' And before you know it you've retreated under your own personal rain cloud.

Laura Berman Fortgang, a coach from the US, talks about finding your essence. Finding your essence means finding a nugget of passion in you that might grow into an ingot of gold. Laura was an actress desperately seeking success. The essence she mined, which ultimately led her to be a professional life coach, was that she loved getting up and performing (which she does now in coaching). Also, she loved understanding people and their motivation (again, she now does this in coaching). Although she wasn't successful as an actress, she found that coaching had many similar roots to acting.

Your clues to your future are in your past. My brother was lucky to find his essence early on. He loved aeroplanes as a kid and would always be scouring the skies identifying types. He was passionate about making model planes from kits and my dad encouraged him all the way. My brother went on to become the aviation editor for a huge specialist magazine and is now a novelist writing about the obvious. You guessed it, planes. Look for your essence in the hobbies and activities that you do in your free time and especially in the careers that you abandoned for being impractical. Start putting together a list of all your passions and establish why you're so enthusiastic about them. Let's say you loved catching bugs and putting them in matchboxes as a child.

What turned you on? Was it being outside? Was it collecting something? Was it the intellectual discipline of collecting bugs of one species? Keep digging until you find that nugget. Don't abandon your dream to play a small game. Play a huge game instead. What have you got to lose?

81
How to love the job you've got

Sometimes you can't have the one you want. So you have to love the one you've got.

One in four of us want to leave our jobs. We can't all do it at once, so here's how to cope until your personal Great Escape.

The bottom line

Hate your job? It's probably for three reasons – you hate the work (it's monotonous or stressful), you hate the environment, including your colleagues, or something else has happened in your life that makes work seem meaningless and you're ready for a lifestyle change. Or it could be that you're in denial. I'm going to come over a bit mystical here, because I firmly believe that sometimes we hate our job because we can't be bothered to address what's really stressing us out in our lives. Our energy is focused elsewhere and until we sort out whatever drama or sadness is soaking up our concentration, we're not likely to find the dream job anytime soon. So the advice here is not about refocusing your CV – there are plenty of other places where you can read up on that. But it will help you relieve stress in the short term and make you feel better about yourself in the long term. And that hopefully will help you raise your energy enough to eventually find another job.

Love your surroundings…

…Just as much as you can. If your workplace is grim and drear, you are not going to feel good. Clear your desk. Sort out clutter. Personalise your work space with objects of beauty and grace. Pin up photos of beautiful vistas you've visited or would like to visit. (It's a bit less personal than family pix.) But whatever you choose to put on your desk, change the visuals every couple of weeks or otherwise your brain stops registering them.

Love your lunchbreaks

A lunchbreak shouldn't be a scramble for bad food and a desultory walk round a shopping mall. Spend time planning. Every lunch hour should involve movement, fresh air, delicious healthy food and at least one work of art. Works of art are easily available for your perusal (art galleries, department stores) and easily transportable (books, CDs). Always, always take an hour to relax at lunch.

Love your colleagues

Tough one. These could well be the reason you hate your job in the first place. If there are people who specifically annoy you, then find a way to deal with them. Your local bookshop is full of manuals that will teach you how. Allow yourself no more than five minutes a day unloading your woes about work colleagues to a trusted friend or partner – not anyone you work with. This is not goody-goody – it's self-preservation. The more you unload your negativity all over the place, the more you are talking yourself into a hole of unhappiness and stress.

Love yourself

Turn up. Work hard. Do better. Lots of people who are unhappy with their work kid themselves that they are working really hard, when in fact their work is shoddy and second-rate. If you're not up to speed, improve your knowledge base and skills. If your work is lazy, look at everything you produce or every service you offer and ask yourself how you can make it special, imbue it with your uniqueness, breathe creativity and a little bit of love into it. Doing every task diligently and with positivity will vastly increase your self-esteem.

Love your dreams

Most of us couldn't have got through school without the ability to drift away on a pleasant reverie of future plans. For five minutes in every hour allow yourself to dream. Read through job pages that aren't related to your present job. You may see a position or course that fires your imagination in a completely new direction.

Boost work morale in a stressful workplace by starting group traditions beyond getting drunk on Friday night and moaning. Go out for a Chinese on pay day or book an awayday at a spa or have a whip-round every birthday and celebrate with champagne and cake.

Workplace support

In the workplace, as employees we have our informal support network of close colleagues, if we are fortunate, which can be a source of helpful advice. Larger employers provide access to counselling through 'Employee Assistance Programmes' or access to occupational health services. A free phone advice and support service is available through the Samaritans. Some people benefit from these services, but in my professional experience, many more people leave it late to get help, perhaps due to the perceived 'stigma' of being seen as not being able to cope. It happens to most of us at some stage in our lives!

The good news is that one of the most potent ways of boosting our coping skills is through talking to a trusted friend or colleague – do not underestimate the value of your personal support network!

82
Meditate on Wellness

Find the space for your mind and meditate on a daily basis.

How many books on meditation do you own? Whether it's twenty-five or none, neither approach will actually get you meditating. The former is only useful if you plan to open a library and doing nothing won't get you anywhere.

We're subject to hundreds of stimuli every day and our reaction to these stimuli can constitute stress. However, we all know that an event we perceive as stressful may not be perceived as stressful to someone else in the same situation. Dr Hans Selye first coined the term 'stress' in the 1950s and it has quickly become an umbrella term for many of the various pressures we experience in life. Some stressors (an event that produces the stress response) are unavoidable, like gravity or exposure to toxic chemicals, while others are purely down to perception – in other words, how you see things will determine how much stress you'll experience. We therefore need to somehow see events differently, through a different pair of glasses. Rose-tinted ones are my personal favourite.

Calming the mind down from stressful thoughts is a powerful way to regain control of uncontrollable events that you could therefore feel anxious about. Meditation has been seen by many as Eastern mystical claptrap. In fact, meditation got a bad press many years ago, as sceptics thought that while there were no thoughts in the mind the devil could nip in and take over.

However, if you've ever actually tried to empty your mind for a moment, you'll have realised that it's virtually impossible, at least for any length of time. Meditation isn't about emptying the mind, it's about observation of the thoughts that are there, like watching clouds drift across a deep blue sky or observing buses travelling down an empty road (at which point you know you must be meditating!). The difference is, you choose not to be pulled down by the thoughts by not giving them any emotional charge. It really is liberating once the penny drops that you are not your thoughts.

There are hundreds of ways to meditate. The simplest is Breath Meditation, which involves sitting quietly observing the breath entering and leaving the body. Then there's Walking Meditation, which is simply observing yourself walking, mindful only of what you're physically doing. Watching the flickering flames of a candle is meditation, as is being absorbed utterly in a hobby. There is even a type of meditation where you concentrate fully on doing the household chores, totally engaged in what you're doing.

To be honest, the easiest way to get into meditation is to throw out all those books and replace them with CDs. There's no way you can read the instructions while attempting to meditate, you'll just get distracted, which defeats the whole point of the meditation experience. So, which method to go for? Go for the relaxation ones to start with. You might not think of these as meditation, but anything that helps concentrate the mind fully is meditation. Recording your own meditation tape works well too, although you might think this is a bit naff.

Body Scan Meditation is also a great one to start with. The first time you do this, tape a script so that next time you can just listen with headphones. Find a comfortable space and lie down, allowing your eyes to gently close. Be aware of your breathing in and out. When you're ready, bring your attention to your left foot and the toes on your foot. Feel like you're breathing into your foot (sounds weird I know). On your script say something like, 'I feel my foot, my foot is relaxed, my foot is completely relaxed.' Work your way up your legs, up through your body and into your head. Don't leave anything out, including the naughty bits! Spend two or three minutes at the end just lying on your back in silence, then bring yourself back to the room. Nice and gently does it. It isn't advisable at this point to dip into the BBC's sound archive and use a klaxon or the *Titanic*'s foghorn, as this will undoubtedly undo that nice relaxed, warm, cuddly feeling. The whole thing should last about 20 minutes or so and practising once a day should really make a difference. And what differences should you expect? Striving for a result is a real no-no in meditation, but between you, me and the gatepost, you should definitely start seeing the world through those rose-coloured specs.

Meditate for calmness

There are hundreds of ways to meditate. The simplest is Breath Meditation, which involves sitting quietly observing the breath entering and leaving the body. Here's your recommended process:

Find a quiet place, away from distractions, sit on a comfortable, upright seat, so your back is supported and your shoulders and arms can relax.

Close your eyes and sense your body in the seat; try to let yourself sink into the seat by letting go, but do not slump. Be aware of your feet on the ground and let your legs relax.

Focus on your breath, starting with the inhalation. Fill up your lungs slowly, feeling the sensations of your breathing.

Pause briefly before letting your breath out, but then gently control the pace of your exhalation. Start the process again in a soft and relaxed manner.

You are on your way! Practise this breathing meditation for 5 to 10 rounds of breathing (inhale and exhale = 1 round), becoming more aware of the sensation of breathing.

Most people feel the calming effect of breathing meditation within 2 to 3 breaths, as it dampens down the cortical arousal (front part of your brain) and reduces the level of stress hormones (cortisol, adrenaline). Your brain can then start its recuperation process.

Resources

Supplements

These are the supplement suppliers I like, which provide high quality nutrition.

Cytoplan: www.cytoplan.co.uk

Wild nutrition: www.wildnutrition.com

Biocare: www.biocare.co.uk, particularly for their probiotic supplements.

BetterYou: betteryou.com, try their Vitamin D spray.

Superfoods: www.superfoodplus.co.uk or www.kiki-health.com

Organic information

Soil Association: www.soilassociation.org

Veg boxes (both do recipe boxes)

Abel and Cole: www.abelandcole.co.uk

Riverford: www.riverford.co.uk

Vegetable wash

Veggi Wash: www.veggiwash.co.uk

Juicers and blenders

Champion juicer: www.championjuicer.com

Other juicers: healthyreturns.co.uk/juicers

Ninja smoothie maker: ninjakitchen.eu/uk/product-category/ products/ninja-personal-blenders

Vitamix blenders: www.vitamix.co.uk

Water filter jugs

Biocera: www.water-for-health.co.uk/alkaline-jug-filters.html

Herbal teas

Yogi tea have a good range, which I've recently been enjoying: www.yogitea.com/en/products

Heart rate monitors: www.polarusa.com or www.heartratemonitor.co.uk

Meal planners

A range is available here: www.paperchase.co.uk/catalogsearch/result/?q=meal+planner

Bike saddles

Swallow saddles: www.brooksengland.com

Sports bras

One of your most important bits of kit if you're a woman: www.boobydoo.co.uk

Mindfulness resources

MindStore: www.mindstore.com

Seasonal affective disorder

Light boxes: www.healthy-house.co.uk/lifestyle/light-therapy-s-a-d

Afterword

Well, did you read the book from cover to cover? I am impressed! Even if you have put one action point from this book into practice it will begin to make a huge impact on your life. We need to fit Wellness into our working lives because we spend a huge amount of time at work. Wellness is not an accident – you need to plan for it.

The major gobbler of good health intention is time so remember to set aside time in your diary for fitness, time to order the food, time to cook the food, much as you would plan a project at work. Don't let your boundaries be eroded by others – it can easily happen. We react to our boss, one more thing to finish off before the weekend, we stay late at work and our good intention to go to the gym evaporates.

Modern technology has made us so reactionary. Remember when we just used to be late for appointments? Someone would wait over an hour without being particularly worried about the other person having been abducted by aliens. We read a book, we relaxed in a café. Even if they didn't show you didn't assume that they had been in a fatal crash over the Atlantic. Nowadays if someone is *one* minute late we are onto it, madly texting or emailing, *WHERE ARE YOU?!!*

So remember that modern technology is a huge drag on our time and Wellness. Switch it off – pour yourself a big glass of water, drop your smartphone in it and breathe – Ahhhh.